THE AORTIC ARCH AND ITS MALFORMATIONS

THE AORTIC ARCH
AND ITS MALFORMATIONS

WITH EMPHASIS ON THE
ANGIOGRAPHIC FEATURES

By

WADE H. SHUFORD, M.D.

Professor of Radiology
Emory University School of Medicine
Director, Division of Diagnostic Roentgenology
Grady Memorial Hospital, Atlanta, Georgia

and

ROBERT G. SYBERS, M.D., Ph.D.

Professor of Radiology
Emory University School of Medicine
Director of Radiology Teaching Program
for Interns and Medical Students
Emory University School of Medicine
and Grady Memorial Hospital
Radiologist, Department of Radiology
Grady Memorial Hospital, Atlanta, Georgia

Medical Illustrations
Grover B. Hogan, B.S., M.S.

Director, Department of Medical Illustration
Emory University School of Medicine
and Grady Memorial Hospital

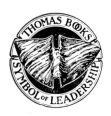

CHARLES C THOMAS · PUBLISHER
Springfield · Illinois · U.S.A.

Published and Distributed Throughout the World by
CHARLES C THOMAS • PUBLISHER
Bannerstone House
301-327 East Lawrence Avenue, Springfield, Illinois, U.S.A.

Library of Congress Catalog Card Number: 73-4017

With THOMAS BOOKS *careful attention is given to all details of
manufacturing and design. It is the Publisher's desire to present books
that are satisfactory as to their physical qualities and artistic possibilities
and appropriate for their particular use.* THOMAS BOOKS *will be true
to those laws of quality that assure a good name and good will.*

Printed in the United States of America
P-4

Library of Congress Cataloging in Publication Data

Shuford, Wade H.
  The aortic arch and its malformations.

  1. Aorta—Abnormalities and deformities. I. Sybers,
Robert G., joint author. II. Title. [DNLM: 1. Aorta—
Abnormalities. 2. Aortography. WG 410 S562a 1973]
RC701.S48   616.1'3   73-4017

ISBN 0-398-02854-0

To Our Families

PREFACE

This book has but one purpose: to provide practical information to physicians who have a specific interest in malformations of the aortic arch. It is intended for use primarily by radiologists. However, this text should prove valuable to medical students, pediatricians, cardiologists, thoracic surgeons and pathologists as well.

It is largely a compilation of our published papers on malformations of the aortic arch. We have been gratified by the response they have received, and judging from the number of requests for reprints, it is apparent that there is considerable interest in this subject. It is for this reason that this material has been put together in book form to make it more readily available to the radiologist.

This monograph reflects our experience with malformations of the aortic arch encountered at Grady Memorial Hospital, a large metropolitan general hospital. We have deliberately selected those anomalies that are important, either because of their radiological features or their clinical manifestations. No attempt has been made to cover all the malformations of the aortic arch that are theoretically possible. These have been thoroughly discussed by Stewart, Kincaid, and Edwards in their *Atlas of Vascular Rings and Related Malformations of the Aortic Arch System*. One malformation, the cervical aortic arch, is described in greater detail than would seem warranted, considering the infrequency with which it is encountered. This has been done so advisedly, but the striking roentgenological findings and the angiographic descriptions of most of the reported cases seem to justify this inclusion.

To a large extent, this text is concerned with the angiographic features of the aortic arch malformations. Material from many sources has been used to illustrate the angiographic findings of the common aortic arch anomalies. In addition, we have included angiograms from some of the more rare arch anomalies which are important in the differential diagnosis.

Also, this book emphasizes the development of the aortic arch malformations. We are indebted to Edwards for his concept of a functioning double aortic arch which is used as the starting point to explain the embryology of the aortic arch. Beginning with a double aortic arch, we have traced the development of the aortic arch malformations through an intermediate stage to the final result. This approach has been proven particularly helpful to radiological residents and medical students in their understanding of the development of the aortic arch. We believe this text will materially supplement information on the aortic arch not readily available in most books of radiology.

W. H. SHUFORD

R. G. SYBERS

ACKNOWLEDGMENTS

WE WOULD LIKE TO EXPRESS our sincere gratitude to Dr. Heinz Stephen Weens, Professor and Chairman, Department of Radiology, Emory University School of Medicine and Grady Memorial Hospital. He provided the stimulus, and it was his suggestion that this book be written.

Many people have contributed to the preparation of this volume. We are especially indebted to Mr. Grover B. Hogan of the Department of Medical Illustration. This book could not have been written without his help. His superb drawings greatly aid the understanding of the embryology of malformations of the aortic arch. At all times he has been most cooperative, and his suggestions have been invaluable.

To the physicians who have so kindly provided us with their published cases, we are most appreciative. Acknowledgment is made in the case report to the contributing author.

The photography was done under the supervision of Mr. Joe Jackson and Mr. Bob Beveridge of the Department of Medical Illustration with assistance from Mr. Eddie Jackson. Mr. Eugene Sedberry of LogEtronics Inc. took some of our difficult angiograms, and provided us with excellent photographic reproductions. Labeling of a number of the x-rays and drawings was performed by Miss Patsy Byran and Mrs. Susan Clark.

Lastly, to Miss Margaret Houser, for her diligent efforts in correcting, typing and retyping the manuscript, we express our sincere thanks.

LIST OF ILLUSTRATIONS

CONTENTS

THE AORTIC ARCH AND ITS MALFORMATIONS

CHAPTER 1

DEVELOPMENTAL BASIS OF THE AORTIC ARCH

AND ITS MALFORMATIONS

To explain the development of the aortic arch and its mal-formations, we have employed Edwards' hypothetical double aortic arch system as a basic pattern from which all aortic arch anomalies may be derived.[4, 5] Figure 1-1 is a diagram of this hypothetical double aortic arch in which there is an aortic arch and a ductus arteriosus on each side. Each aortic arch gives rise to a common carotid and a subclavian artery. The descending aorta is in the midline. Interruption of this arch system at different locations can explain the development of the normal aortic arch and the aortic arch anomalies.[2, 4, 5]

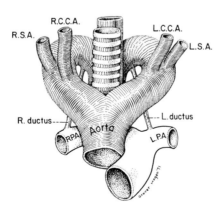

Figure 1-1. Diagram of Edwards' hypothetical double aortic arch system showing bilateral aortic arches and bilateral ductus arteriosi.

3

Derivation of the Hypothetical Double Aortic Arch

The stages in the development of this hypothetical double aortic arch system utilizing the Rathke diagram are shown in the following illustrations (Figs. 1-2 through 1-8).

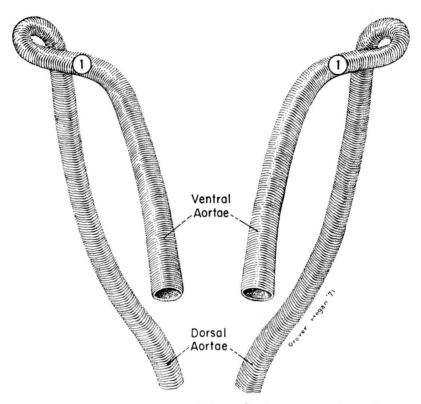

Figure 1-2. Two primitive ventral (ascending) aortae continue via symmetrical aortic arches into descending primitive aortae.[1, 3]

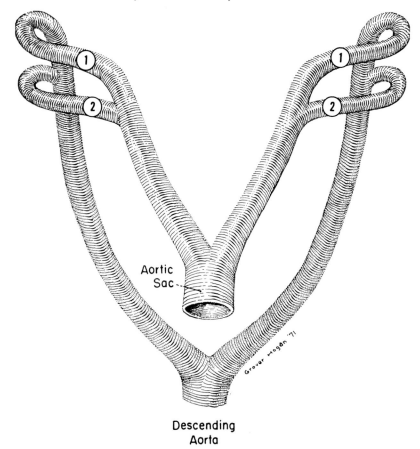

Descending Aorta

Figure 1-3. The proximal portions of the ventral aortae fuse to form a single midline trunk—the aortic sac. The paired dorsal aortae fuse to form a midline descending aorta. Between the ventral and dorsal aortae, the first two pairs of symmetrical branchial aortic arches develop.[1, 3, 4]

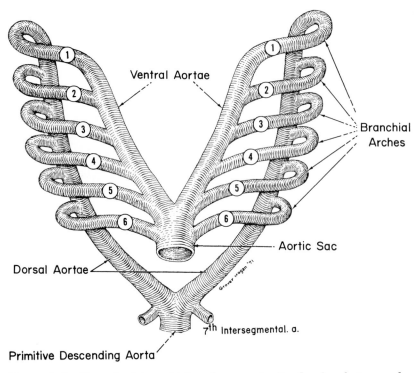

Figure 1-4. Six paired branchial arches eventually develop between the dorsal and ventral aortae forming the basic Rathke diagram.[3, 4]

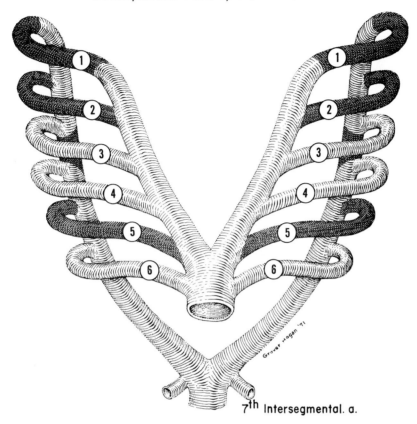

7th Intersegmental. a.

Figure 1-5. Although there are six pairs of primitive branchial arches, all are not present at any one time. The first two arches disappear once the third and fourth branchial arches are established. The fifth arch appears and quickly regresses as do also those parts of the primitive dorsal aortae between the third and fourth arches bilaterally. The sixth arch persists. The seventh intersegmental arteries develop from the dorsal aortae.[1, 3] The shaded areas represent the segments of regression.

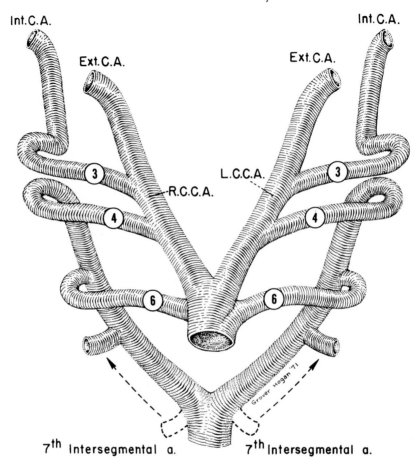

Figure 1-6. As the branchial arches are developing and regressing, changes occur in the aortic sac. This is divided into an aortic and pulmonary portion. The pulmonary portion becomes the pulmonary trunk and the aortic portion subsequently becomes the ascending aorta. The right and left third arches and dorsal aortae cephalad to these arches becomes the right and left internal carotid arteries. The ventral aortae cephalad to these arches become the right and left external carotid arteries. The fourth branchial arches form the aortic arches. The fifth branchial arches regress early in development. The sixth branchial arches persist to eventually form the pulmonary arteries and ductus arteriosi. The seventh intersegmental arteries arising from the dorsal aorta migrate cephalad with the caudal migration of the heart.[1, 3]

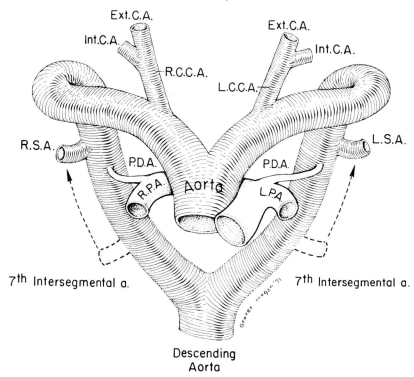

Figure 1-7. A primitive double aortic arch is formed in which there is an aortic arch and a ductus arteriosus on each side. The descending aorta is in the midline. From each of the two aortic arches arise a common carotid artery and a subclavian artery as independent branches.[5] The ventral portions of the sixth branchial arches form the pulmonary arteries and the dorsal segments of the sixth branchial arches become the ductus arteriosi. The seventh intersegmental arteries assume a position between the ductus arteriosi and the common carotid arteries, and become the subclavian arteries.[2, 3]

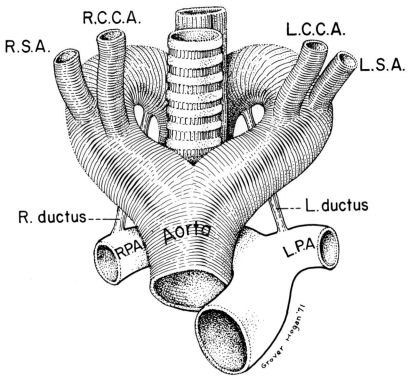

Figure 1-8. This hypothetical double aortic arch completely encircles the trachea and esophagus forming a vascular ring.

REFERENCES

1. Barry, Alexander: Aortic arch derivatives in the human adult. *Anat Rec,* *111*:221, 1951.
2. Blake, H. A., and Manion, W. C.: Thoracic arterial arch anomalies. *Circulation, 26*:251, 1962.
3. Congdon, E. D.: Transformation of the aortic arch system during the development of the human embryo. *Contrib Embryol, 14*:47, 1922.
4. Edwards, J. E.: Anomalies of the derivatives of the aortic arch system. *Med Clin North Am, 32*:925, 1948.
5. Stewart, J. R.; Kincaid, O. W., and Edwards, J. E.: *An Atlas of Vascular Rings and Related Malformations of the Aortic Arch System.* Springfield, Thomas, 1964, pp. 3-9.

CHAPTER 2

THE NORMAL LEFT AORTIC ARCH

Definition. The normal left aortic arch begins as a continuation of the ascending aorta. It passes anteriorly and to the left of the trachea and esophagus and continues as the descending aorta on the left side of the spine.[4] Attached to the inner aspect of the left arch is the ligamentum arteriosum (obliterated ductus arteriosus).

Development. Using Edwards' hypothetical double aortic arch system as the embryologic starting point, the normal left aortic arch results from interruption of the dorsal segment of the embryonic right arch between the right subclavian artery and the descending aorta with regression of the right ductus arteriosus (Fig. 2-1).[1] The midline dorsal aorta shifts to the left of the spine to become the descending aorta. This shift is due to the

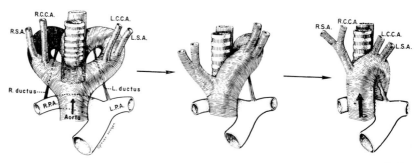

Figure 2-1. Development of left aortic arch. There is interruption of the right embryonic arch in the hypothetical double arch between the right subclavian artery and descending aorta. Area in black indicates site of interruption.

12

midline appearance of the vertebral bodies with subsequent displacement of the dorsal aorta.[1]

Chest Roentgenography. The upper border of the cardiovascular shadow, on the left side, is formed by the distal aortic arch as it curves posteriorly to become the descending aorta. This presents as a localized convexity—the aortic knob—just below the left clavicle and above the left tracheobronchial angle.[2] The aortic arch usually produces a lateral indentation on the opacified esophagus and slightly deviates the trachea to the right.

Angiographic Features. Contrast studies show the thoracic aorta to arch to the left side. The branches of the aortic arch are the innominate (brachiocephalic), the left common carotid and the left subclavian arteries.[4] This is the most common pattern occurring in 70 percent of patients. In approximately 25 percent of patients, the innominate and the left common carotid arteries arise from a common trunk.[4]

Not infrequently, the normal left aortic arch shows a diverticulum-like structure arising from the medial aspect of the left arch distal to the origin of the left subclavian artery (Fig. 2-2).[3] This diverticulum represents persistence of the most distal portion of the embryonic right arch (Fig. 2-3).[3] While this diverticulum is in anatomic proximity to the left ductus arteriosus, it is not the result of traction by the left ductus arteriosus.

REFERENCES

1. Edwards, J. E.: Anomalies of the derivatives of the aortic arch system. *Med Clin North Am, 32*:925, 1948.
2. Elliott, L. P., and Schiebler, G. L.: *X-Ray Diagnosis of Congential Cardiac Disease.* Springfield, Thomas, 1968, pp. 8-11, 33-36.
3. Grollman, J. H., Jr.; Paris, C. H., and Hamilton, L. C.: Congenital diverticula of the aortic arch. *N Engl J Med, 276*:1178, 1967.
4. Oelrich, T. M.: The cardiovascular system. In Henry Morris: *Human Anatomy: A Complete Systematic Treatise.* Edited by B. J. Anson. 12th ed. New York, Blakiston Co., 1966, pp. 667-670.

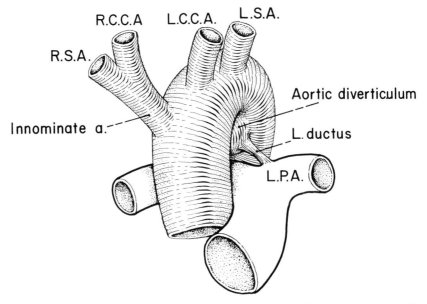

Figure 2-2. Left aortic arch and diverticulum arising from inner aspect of distal arch.

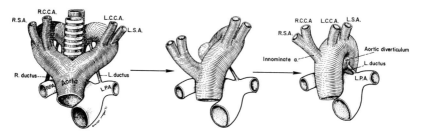

Figure 2-3. Development of left aortic arch and aortic diverticulum. There has been interruption of the embryonic right arch in the hypothetical double aortic arch between the right subclavian artery and descending aorta. The most distal portion of the embryonic right arch persists forming an aortic diverticulum. The right ductus arteriosus regresses. Area in black indicates site of interruption.

Representative Cases

Case 1. Patient with gunshot injury of chest.

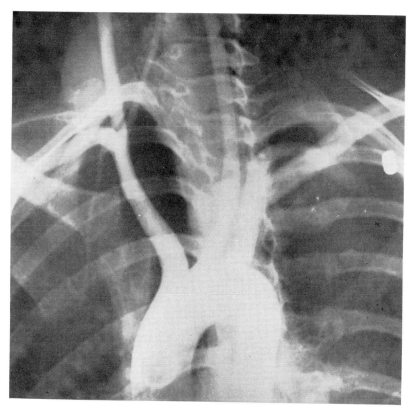

Figure 2-4. Case 1. Normal left arch. Left anterior projection. The innominate artery is the first branch followed by the left common carotid and the left subclavian arteries.

Representative Cases

Case 2. Child with patent ductus arteriosus.

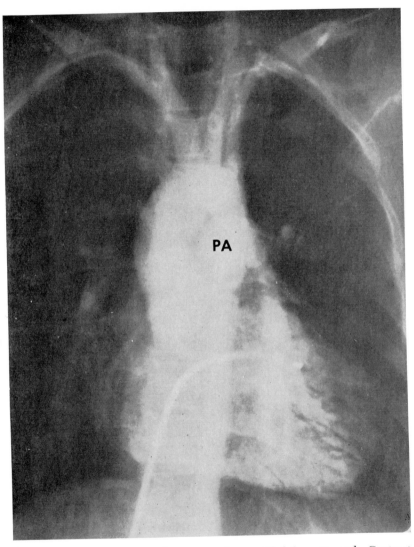

Figure 2-5. Case 2. Patent ductus arteriosus with left aortic arch. Contrast media injected into left ventricle. With opacification of the aorta, there is immediate filling of pulmonary circulation through a patent ductus arteriosus. The first branch of the arch is the innominate artery followed by the left common carotid and the left subclavian arteries. PA = pulmonary artery.

Case 3. Sixty-year-old man with cerebrovascular accident.

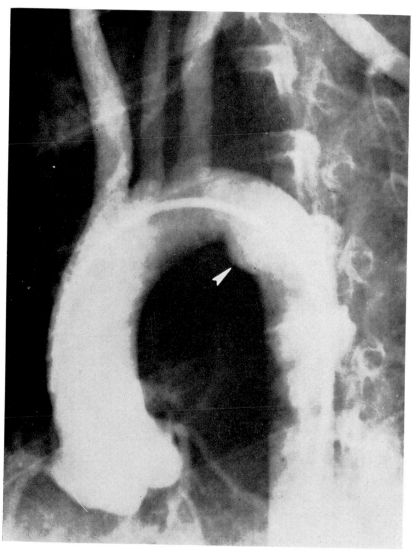

Figure 2-6. Case 3. Normal left arch with aortic diverticulum. Aortogram in right posterior oblique projection. Arrow points to diverticulum along concavity of aortic arch distal to left subclavian artery. This structure represents a remnant of the most distal portion of the embryonic right arch (Fig. 2-3).

CHAPTER 3

LEFT AORTIC ARCH WITH ABERRANT RIGHT

SUBCLAVIAN ARTERY

Definition. The first branch of the left aortic arch is the right common carotid artery, followed by the left common carotid artery and the left subclavian artery in that order. The right subclavian artery arises as the fourth branch from the distal left arch, crossing behind the esophagus and extending obliquely upward to the right arm. [2,6] The aorta descends on the left side (Fig. 3-1).

Incidence and Clinical Significance. Left aortic arch with an aberrant right subclavian artery is the most common malformation of the aortic arch. Approximately one person in two hundred has this anomaly.[2] It may be observed during routine barium study of the esophagus. Almost never does this malformation produce dysphagia or respiratory symptoms, and these patients are not studied by angiography.[1] In study of patients with congenital heart disease, particularly coarctation of the aorta and tetrology of Fallot, one occasionally encounters a left aortic arch with an aberrant right subclavian artery.[7]

When an aberrant right subclavian artery is associated with coarctation of the aorta, the origin of the aberrant subclavian vessel in relation to the coarctate segment may be important. If the aberrant right subclavian artery arises distal to the site of coarctation, the right subclavian artery is a low pressure artery, and there may be a large retrograde flow through this vessel to

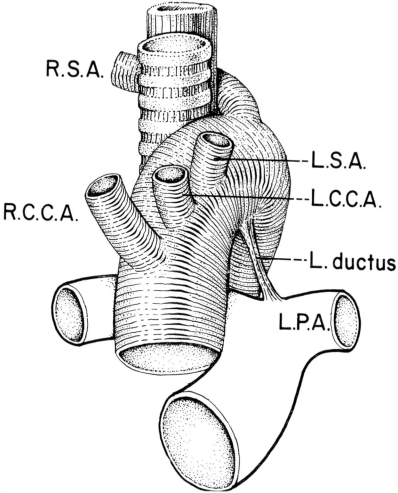

R.S.A.

L.S.A.

L.C.C.A.

R.C.C.A.

L. ductus

L.P.A.

Figure 3-1. Left aortic arch with aberrant right subclavian artery. The right subclavian artery is the fourth branch of the aortic arch and passes behind the esophagus to reach the right arm.

the descending aorta. (See Chapter 11, Fig. 11-11 *A, B, C, D;* Fig. 11-12 *A, B, C;* and Fig. 11-13.) Under these circumstances the usual collateral pathways do not develop on the right side, and rib notching occurs on the left side only. If the origin of the aberrant right subclavian artery is proximal to the coarctation, blood flow in the aberrant vessel is in the normal direction (Fig.

11-10). In these patients rib notching may be present on both sides.

Development. This abnormality results from interruption of the right arch in the hypothetical double aortic arch pattern between the right common carotid and right subclavian arteries. The right ductus arteriosus usually disappears (Fig. 3-2).[7]

The right subclavian artery may originate from a diverticulum-like structure of the aorta (diverticulum of Kommerell), which represents persistence of the most distal portion of the embryonic right arch (Fig. 3-3).[3, 5]

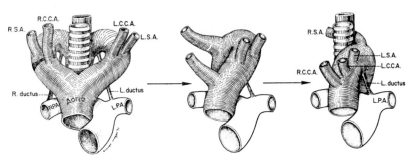

Figure 3-2. Development of left aortic arch with aberrant right subclavian artery. There is interruption of the right embryonic arch in the hypothetical double aortic arch between the right common carotid and right subclavian arteries. The right ductus disappears. Area in black indicates site of interruption.

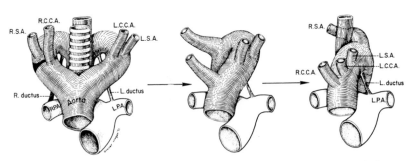

Figure 3-3. Development of left aortic arch with aberrant right subclavian artery arising from an aortic diverticulum. There is interruption of the embryonic right arch in the hypothetical double aortic arch between the right common carotid and right subclavian arteries. The distal portion of the embryonic right arch persists and gives origin to the right subclavian artery. Area in black indicates site of interruption.

Chest Roentgenography. The plain chest roentgenogram in all of our patients has been normal. However, the anomalous vessel itself may be visible.[7] In a few reported cases, the diverticulum-like origin of the aberrant vessel produced a convex prominence just above the aortic knob simulating a mediastinal tumor.[1, 4, 5]

Barium studies of the esophagus reveal a finger-sized posterior compression defect on the esophagus running obliquely upward from left to right.[2]

Angiographic Features. Angiography shows a left aortic arch. The aberrant right subclavian artery originates at the junction of the distal arch and upper descending aorta and courses upward and obliquely to the right arm.[7] Occasionally, an aortic diverticulum is present at the origin of the right subclavian artery from the aorta.[4]

REFERENCES

1. Felson, B.; Cohen, S.; Courter, S. R., and McGuire, J.: Anomalous right subclavian artery. *Radiology*, 54:340, 1950.
2. Klinkhamer, A. C.: *Esophagography in Anomalies of the Aortic Arch System.* Baltimore, Williams & Wilkins, 1969, pp. 16-30.
3. Kommerell, B.: Verlagerung des Osophagus durch eine abnorm verlaufende Ateria sublcavia dextra (ateria lusoria). *Fortschr Geb Roentgenstr Nuklearmed*, 54:590-595, 1936.
4. Richards, W. C. D., and Elliott, C. E.: Aneurysm of an anomalous right subclavian artery. *Br Heart*, 19:191, 1957.
5. Shannon, J. M.: Aberrant right subclavian artery with Kommerell's diverticulum. *J. Thorac Cardiovasc Surg*, 41:408, 1961.
6. Stauffer, H. M., and Pote, H. H.: Anomalous right subclivian artery originating on left as last branch of aortic arch. *Am J Roentgenol Radium Ther Nucl Med*, 56:13, 1946.
7. Stewart, J. R.; Kincaid, O. W., and Edwards, J. E.: *An Atlas of Vascular Rings and Related Malformations of the Aortic Arch System.* Springfield, Thomas, 1964, pp. 52-60.

Representative Cases

Case 1. This six-year-old child was referred to the Heart Clinic because of a functional murmur. There was no symptoms of heart disease, dysphagia, choking sensations or vomiting. Chest roentgenogram (Fig. 3-4 A) was negative. The findings illustrated on the esophagogram (Fig. 3-4 B) are typical of an aberrant right subclavian artery.

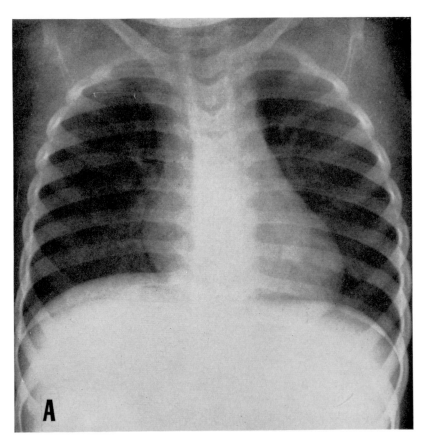

Figure 3-4 A. Case 1. Left aortic arch with aberrant right subclavian artery. Chest x-ray is negative. On rare occasions, the shadow cast by this vessel may be visible on the frontal chest roentgenogram.

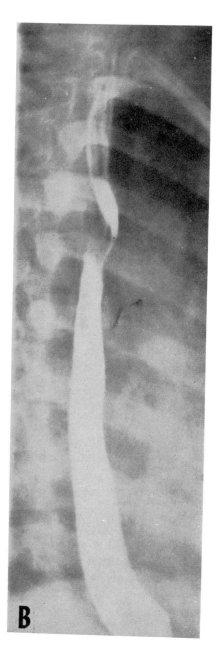

Figure 3-4 (B). Case 1. Left aortic arch with aberrant right subclavian artery. Esophagogram in right anterior oblique projection. The aberrant right subclavian artery produces an oblique indentation on the posterior esophageal wall at the level of T-4-5 running upward from left to right.

Representative Cases

Case 2. Left arch with aberrant right subclavian artery in a six-month-old child with double-outlet right ventricle. There was no difficulty swallowing. Selective right ventriculograms (Fig. 3-5) show anomalous origin of the right subclavian artery as the fourth branch of the aortic arch.

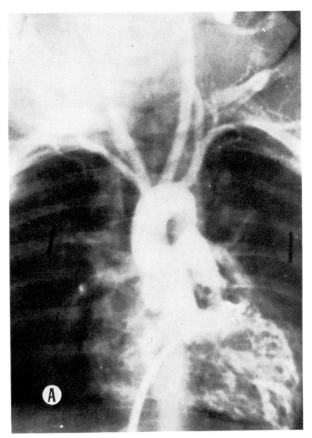

Figure 3-5 A. Case 2. Double-outlet right ventricle with left aortic arch and aberrant right subclavian artery. Frontal selective right ventriculogram (A) shows simultaneous visualization of the aorta and pulmonary artery. The aberrant right subclavian artery arises as the fourth branch from the distal aortic arch.

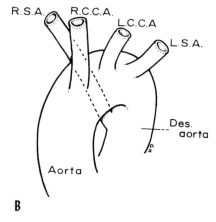

B

Figure 3-5 B. Diagram of frontal angiogram.

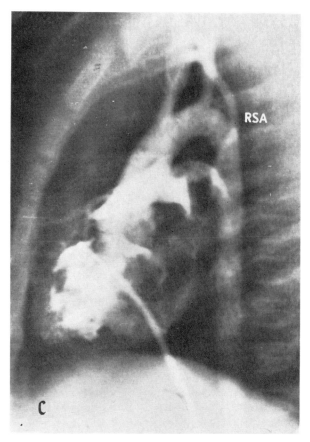

Figure 3-5 C. Lateral ventriculogram showing aberrant origin of right subclavian artery. RSA = right subclavian artery.

Representative Cases

Case 3.   Persistent truncus arteriosus with left arch and aberrant right subclavian artery. Barium studies of the esophagus reveal characteristic posterior compression defect of a retroesophageal vessel (Fig. 3-6 *A* & *B*). Right ventriculogram (Fig. 3-6 *C* & *D*) shows anomalous course of the right subclavian artery.

At autopsy, the right pulmonary artery arose from the posterior portion of the aortic arch and coursed downward behind the right main bronchus to enter the hilum of the right lung. From the upper descending aorta, a large bronchial artery supplied the left lung.

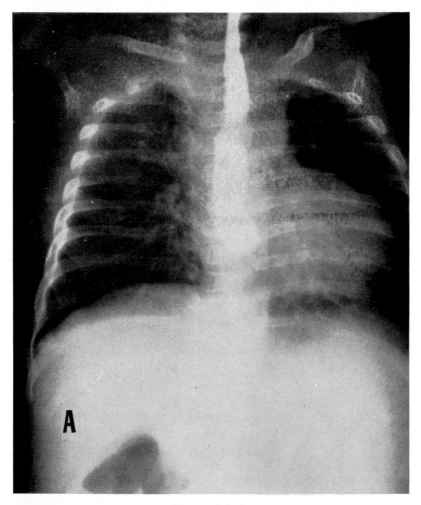

Figure 3-6 A,

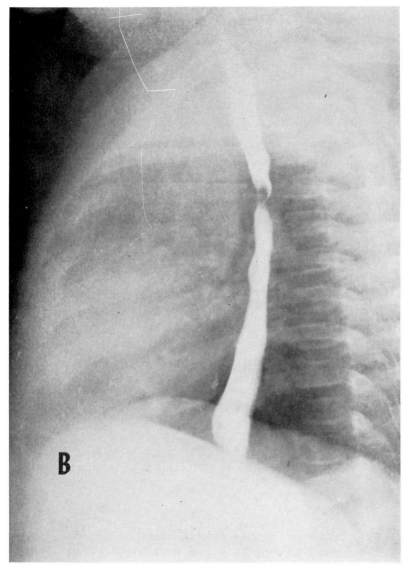

Figure 3-6. Case 3. Persistent truncus with left aortic arch and aberrant right subclavian artery. Frontal and lateral esophagograms (*A & B*) reveal an oblique retroesophageal compression defect on the contrast-filled esophagus at the level of the aortic arch.

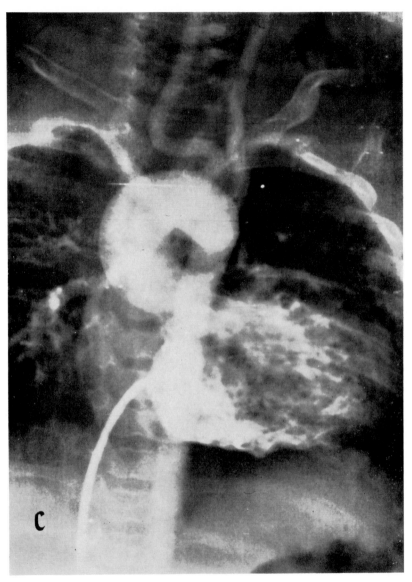

Figure 3-6. Case 3. Persistent truncus with left aortic arch and aberrant right subclavian artery. Right ventriculogram (C) reveals a single arterial trunk arising from both ventricles. The first branch of the arch is the right common carotid artery, followed by the left common carotid artery and the left subclavian artery. The right subclavian artery arises from the upper descending aorta as the fourth branch.

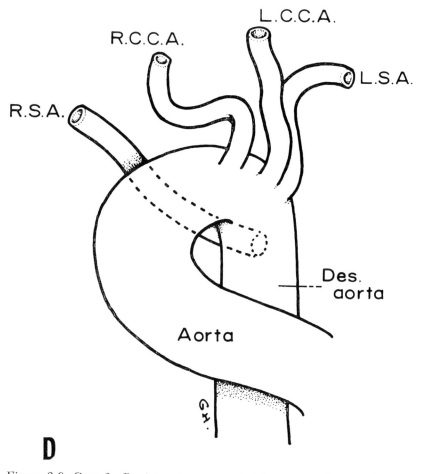

Figure 3-6. Case 3. Persistent truncus with left aortic arch and aberrant right subclavian artery. (*D*) Diagram of frontal angiogram.

CHAPTER 4

LEFT AORTIC ARCH WITH RIGHT

DESCENDING AORTA

Definition. This anomaly is often referred to as left aortic arch (posterior or circumflex type) with right descending aorta.[3] The left aortic arch arises from the ascending aorta and passes backward to the left of the trachea and esophagus. The terminal portion of the aortic arch crosses to the right side of the mediastinum behind the esophagus, turning abruptly downward, to continue as the right descending aorta.[5]

Incidence and Clinical Significance. Only a few cases with this malformation have been reported.[1, 2, 3, 4, 5, 6] The two patients reported by Paul were associated with tetralogy of Fallot.[5] Edwards' case of left aortic arch and right descending aorta with an aberrant origin of the right subclavian artery and a persistent right ligamentum arteriosum resulted in a vascular ring.[2] In three patients reported by Hastreiter, et al., aortic stenosis and tetralogy of Fallot were observed in two. In the other, there was no cardiac defect.[3] In our case, extralobar pulmonary sequestration with venous drainage to the portal vein was associated with this malformation (Figs. 4-1 through 4-5).[6]

Development. In those cases of left aortic arch with right descending aorta and normal branching of the arch vessels, there is interruption of the embryonic right arch in the hypothetical double aortic arch between the right subclavian artery and descending aorta (Fig. 2-1).[7] When the right subclavian artery

30

arises as the fourth branch in patients with left aortic arch and right descending aorta, the development is the same as left aortic arch with aberrant right subclavian artery (Fig. 3-2). The reason for the descent of the upper thoracic aorta to the right of the thoracic spine in these cases is not clear.[3,5]

Chest Roentgenography. On the frontal chest x-ray, the aortic knob is on the left side. There may be absence of the aortic shadow between the aortic knob and upper left border of the heart.[5] The descending aorta may be visualized to the right of the midline.[5] The heart may be enlarged in those patients with an associated cardiac malformation.

Barium studies show the esophagus to be indented on its left margin by the arch of the aorta.[3] The esophagus may descend abnormally to the left of the midline.[6] The descending aorta lies abnormally to the right of the esophagus. At fluoroscopy, a constant finding is a large pulsating posterior compression defect on the barium-filled esophagus representing the retroesophageal portion of the aorta as it crosses from the left side of the spine to descend on the right.[3,6]

The barium esophagogram in this unusual malformation may be indistinguishable from that observed in double aortic arch and right aortic arch with an aberrant left subclavian artery, however, contrast studies of the aorta will readily identify this anomaly.

Angiographic Features. Angiography shows a left aortic arch. Usually the first branch is the innominate artery followed by the left common carotid artery and the left subclavian artery.[6] The right subclavian artery may arise aberrantly as the fourth branch of the left arch.[2] The upper left thoracic aorta crosses the midline to descend on the right.[6]

REFERENCES

1. de Balsac, R. Heim: Left aortic arch (posterior or circumflex type) with right descending aorta. *Am J Cardiol*, 5:546, 1960.
2. Edwards, Jesse E.: Retro-esophageal segment of the left aortic arch, right ligamentum arteriosum and right descending aorta causing a congenital vascular ring about the trachea and esophagus. *Mayo Clin Proc*, 23:108, 1948.
3. Hastreiter, A. R.; d'Cruz, I. A., et al.: Right-sided aorta. II. Right aortic

arch, right descending aorta, and associated anomalies. *Br Heart J,*
28:722, 1966.

4. Heinrich, W. D., and Tamayo, R. P.: Left aortic arch and right descending aorta. A case report. *Am J Roentgenol Radium Ther Nucl
   med,* 76:762, 1956.

5. Paul, R. N.: A new anomaly of the aorta. Left aortic arch with right
   descending aorta. *J Pediatr,* 32:19, 1948.

6. Shuford, W. H., and Sybers, R. G.: Bronchopulmonary sequestration
   with venous drainage to the portal vein. *Am J Roentgenol Radium
   Ther Nucl Med,* 92:547, 1964.

7. Shuford, W. H.; Sybers, R. G., and Edwards, F. K.: The three types
   of right aortic arch. *Am J Roentgenol Radium Ther Nucl Med, 109:*
   67, 1970.

Representative Cases

Case 1. Left aortic arch and right descending aorta associated with
extralobar pulmonary sequestration.

This six-year-old child had repeated bouts of pneumonia. There
was no history to suggest heart disease. Chest x-ray (Fig. 4-1 *A* and
B) showed a homogeneous airless mass in the left lower lobe visible
through the left heart shadow. The heart was of normal size and
configuration. The shadow of the descending aorta was to the right
of the spine. A tentative diagnosis of bronchopulmonary sequestration was made.

Bronchography (Fig. 4-2) showed displacement and crowding of
the segmental bronchi of the left lower lobe by the mass density. No
communication with the tracheo-bronchial tree was evident.

On barium swallow, the middle third of the esophagus was displaced forward and to the right (Fig. 4-3 *A* & *B*).

The course of the thoracic aorta was of interest (Fig. 4-4). The
aortic arch was left-sided. The terminal portion of the arch crossed
the midline to descend on the right side of the spine. The branching
of the arch vessels was normal.

Catheter aortography (Fig. 4-5 *A* & *B*) confirmed the diagnosis
of pulmonary sequestration. An aberrant artery arising from the ab-
dominal aorta at the level of the celiac axis supplied the pulmonary
mass. The venous drainage was to the portal vein.

Surgical exploration revealed an extralobar type of pulmonary
sequestration with the sequestered lung enclosed in its own pleura
in the left lower chest. A large vein drained the mass and emptied
into the portal system.

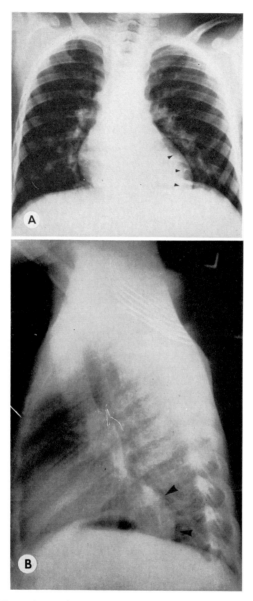

Figure 4-1. Case 1. Left aortic arch and right descending aorta with bronchopulmonary sequestration. (A) An area of increased density (arrows) representing the airless pulmonary mass is visible through the left heart shadow. (B) Arrows show the homogeneous mass to occupy the region of the basilar segments of the left lower lobe. (From W. H. Shuford, and R. G. Sybers: Bronchopulmonary sequestration with venous drainage to the portal veins. *Am J Roentgenol Radium Ther Nucl Med, 106*:118, 1969.)

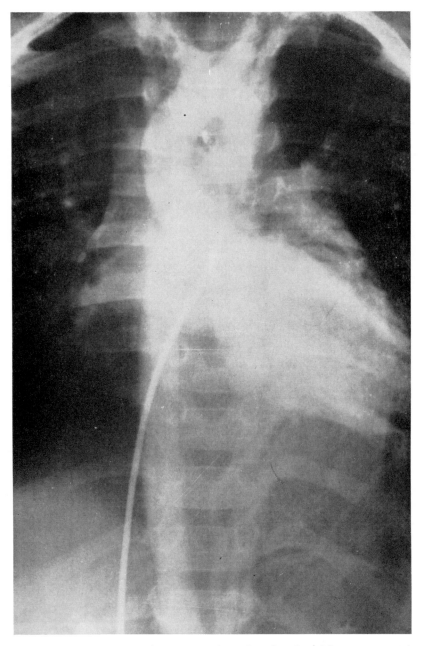

Figure 4-4. Case 1. Left aortic arch and right descending aorta with bronchopulmonary sequestration. Levoangiocardiogram shows a left aortic arch. There is normal branching of the arch vessels. The terminal portion of the aortic arch crosses the midline behind the esophagus to descend on the right side of the spine.

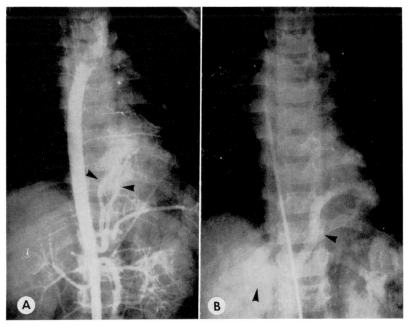

Figure 4-5. Case 1. Left aortic arch and right descending aorta with bronchopulmonary sequestration. (A) Aortogram shows a large aberrant artery from the aorta supplying the sequestered pulmonary tissue through several branches (arrows). (B) Upper arrow indicates a large drainage vein emptying into the portal system (lower arrow). (From W. H. Shuford, and R. G. Sybers: Bronchopulmonary sequestration with venous drainage to the portal veins. *Am J Roentgenol Radium Ther Nucl Med, 105*:118, 1969.)

Representative Cases

Case 2. Left aortic arch with right descending aorta and pulmonic stenosis and a ventricular septal defect. This eight-year-old-girl gave no symptoms of esophageal or tracheal compression.

Chest roentgenogram with the esophagus barium-filled and selective angiocardiograms are shown in Figures 4-6 *A-C* and 4.7. (Courtesy of Dr. Alois R. Hastreiter).

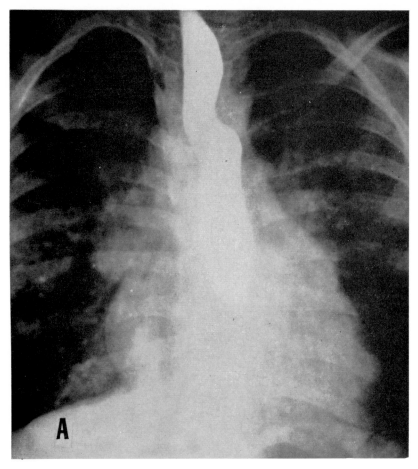

Figure 4-6.   Case 2.   Left aortic arch and right descending aorta. Barium studies of the esophagus. Frontal view (*A*) shows an indentation on the left side of the esophagus at the level of the aortic arch. The distal esophagus is slightly displaced to the left by the right-sided descending aorta.

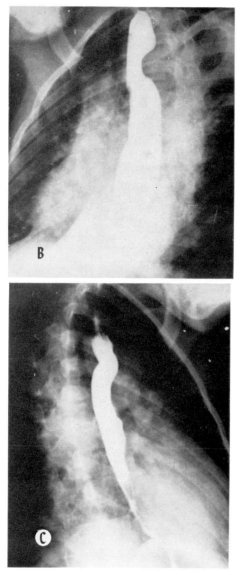

Figure 4-6 (*B* and *C*). Oblique views reveal a posterior compression defect on the barium-filled esophagus produced by the retroesophageal portion of the aorta as it crosses the spinal colum to descend on the right side. (From A. R. Hastreiter, I. A. d'Cruz, and T. Cantez: Right-sided aorta. II. Right aortic arch, right descending aorta, and associated anomalies. *Br Heart J,* 28:722, 1966.)

Representative Cases

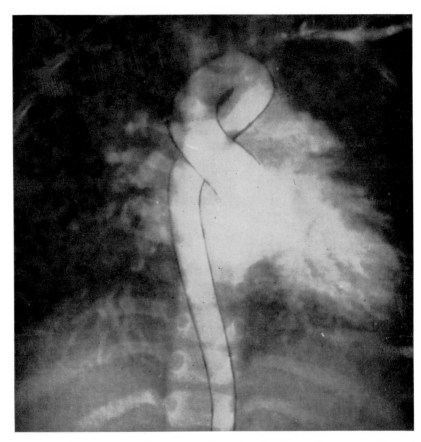

Figure 4-7. Case 2. Left aortic arch and right descending aorta. Frontal levoangiocardiogram reveals a normal ascending aorta. The distal portion of the left arch crosses the mediastinum abruptly to descend on the right side of the spine. (From A. R. Hastreiter, I. A. d'Cruz, and T. Cantez: Right-sided aorta. II. Right aortic arch, right descending aorta, and associated anomalies. *Br Heart J,* 28:722, 1966.)

CHAPTER 5

RIGHT AORTIC ARCH

Definition. The aorta arches to the right of the trachea and esophagus and continues as the upper thoracic aorta to descend either to the right or left of the spine.[3, 5, 10, 26]

Classification. We have classified right aortic arch into types depending upon the branching of the arch vessels. The arrangement of the arch vessels is determined by the location at which the left arch interrupts. Interruption may be in one of four locations in the embryonic left arch in the hypothetical double aortic arch. These sites of interruption are illustrated in Figure 5-1.

TYPES OF RIGHT AORTIC ARCH

Type 1 Right Aortic Arch (mirror-image branching—common type). Interruption occurs in the embryonic left arch in the hypothetical double aortic arch between the left ductus arteriosus and descending aorta.

Type 2 Right Aortic Arch (mirror-image branching—rare type). Interruption occurs in the embryonic left arch in the hypothetical double aortic arch between the left subclavian artery and left ductus arteriosus.

Type 3 Right Aortic Arch (aberrant left subclavian artery). Interruption is between the left common carotid artery and the left subclavian artery in the embryonic left arch.

Type 4 Right Aortic Arch (aberrant left innominate artery). There is interruption in the anterior portion of the embryonic left arch proximal to the origin of the left common carotid artery.

Type 5 Right Aortic Arch (isolation of the left subclavian

41

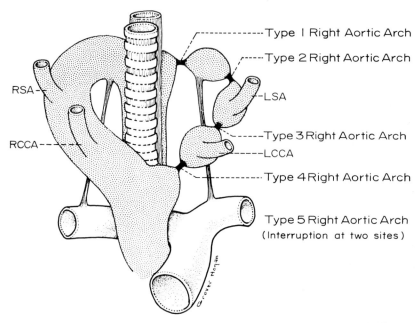

Figure 5-1. Diagram showing sites in the embryonic left arch in the hypothetical double aortic arch where interruption results in the different types
of right aortic arch. In Type 1 right aortic arch (mirror-image branching—
common type) interruption is between the left ductus arteriosus and descending aorta. In Type 2 right aortic arch (mirror-image branching—rare
type) interruption occurs between the left subclavian artery and left ductus arteriosus. Type 3 right aortic arch (aberrant left subclavian artery)
results from interruption between the left common carotid and the left
subclavian artery. In Type 4 right aortic arch (aberrant left innominate
artery) the interruption is proximal to the left common carotid artery. In
Type 5 right aortic arch (isolation of the left subclavian artery) interruption is at two sites: between the left common carotid and left subclavian
arteries and also distal to the left subclavian artery.

artery). Interruption of the embryonic left arch occurs at two
sites.

Theoretically, each of these types may have either a right,
left or bilateral ductus arteriosi [25] In the vast majority of cases, it
is the left ductus arteriosus that persists.[25] Right aortic arch with
only a right ductus arteriosus does not produce a vascular ring.[25,
26] Therefore, we will limit our discussion to right aortic arch
with persistence of the left ductus arteriosus only.

Type 1 Right Aortic Arch
(Mirror-image Branching—Common Type)

Definition. In this type (Fig. 5-2) the right aortic arch has three branches—namely, a left innominate, a right common carotid and a right subclavian artery in that order.[22, 25] The left innominate artery courses anteriorly to the trachea and gives rise to the left common carotid artery and the left subclavian artery. The left ductus arteriosus connects the subclavian portion of the innominate artery to the left pulmonary artery. The aorta arches to the right of the trachea and esophagus, and descends on the right of the spine. We have not encountered a right aortic arch with mirror-image branching in which the aorta descended to the left side of the spine.

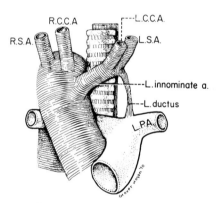

Figure 5-2. Type 1 right aortic arch with mirror-image branching (common type). The first branch of the right arch is the left innominate artery followed by the right common carotid and right subclavian arteries. There is no retroesophageal compression.

Clinical Significance. This type of right aortic arch is almost always associated with cyanotic heart disease, particularly tetralogy of Fallot and truncus arteriosus, and less commonly tricuspid atresia.[25] About 25 percent of patients with tetralogy of Fallot will have a right aortic arch.[5] Of these patients, approximately 90 percent will have mirror-image branching of the arch vessels.[7] The remaining 10 percent will have an aberrant left subclavian artery.[7]

In this type, the right aortic arch is to the right of the trachea and esophagus.[25] The left innominate artery courses anteriorly to the trachea, and the left ductus arteriosus connects the subclavian portion of the innominate artery to the left pulmonary artery. As a result, there is no retroesophageal component and the esophagus is not compressed from behind. These patients do not have symptoms of a vascular ring.[3]

Development. This type results from interruption of the embryonic left arch in the hypothetical double aortic arch between the descending aorta and the left ductus arteriosus. The right ductus arteriosus usually disappears (Fig. 5-3).[10, 22, 25]

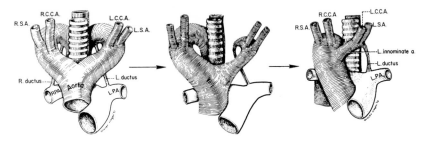

Figure 5-3. Development of Type 1 right aortic arch with mirror-image branching of the arch vessels and a left ductus arteriosus connecting the pulmonary artery to the left subclavian artery. There has been interruption of the embryonic left arch in the hypothetical double aortic arch between the left ductus arteriosus and descending aorta in the area indicated in black. There is no vascular ring present.

Chest Roentgenography. The aortic knob is usually identified along the right border of the mediastinum displacing the superior vena cava to the right.[10] Occasionally the aortic knob is concealed within the shadow of the superior vena cava.[3] When the aortic knob is not visualized, a right aortic arch may be suspected by an indentation on the right side of the trachea. Visualization of the esophagus aids in the diagnosis for the aorta displaces the esophagus to the left.[3, 5] The descending aorta is to the right of the spine.

This malformation does not produce a vascular ring and there is no posterior compression defect on the lateral esophagogram.

Angiographic Features. The ascending aorta courses upward obliquely to the right of the trachea and descends sharply to the right of the midline. The first branch of the right arch is the left innominate artery followed by the right common carotid artery and the right subclavian artery.

Representative Cases

Case 1. Type 1 Right Aortic Arch. Twenty-year-old woman with tetralogy of Fallot.

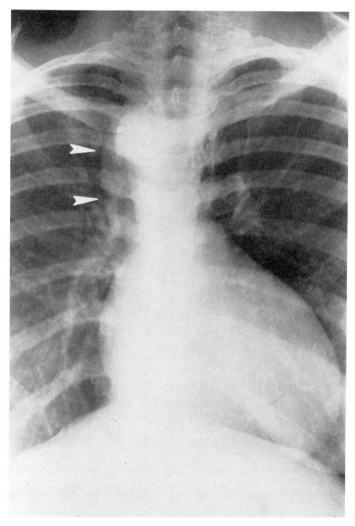

Figure 5-4. Case 1. Tetralogy of Fallot. The aortic knob is visible along the right border of the mediastinum slightly indenting the tracheal air shadow. The superior vena cava (arrows) is displaced to the right. The descending aorta is right-sided. The heart shows right ventricular enlargement.

Representative Cases

Case 2. Type 1 Right Aortic Arch. Four-year-old child with tetralogy of Fallot. Chest roentgenograms (Fig. 5-5 *A* & *B*) show enlargement of the apex of the heart and flattening of the pulmonary artery segment. The pulmonary vasculature is decreased. A right aortic arch indents the right side of the trachea. The lateral view of the esophagus filled with barium reveals no vascular structure compressing the posterior wall of the esophagus.

Angiography (Fig. 5-5 *C* & *D*) confirms the presence of right aortic arch. The first branch of the right arch is the left innominate artery, and the right common carotid and right subclavian arteries arise as the second and third branches. The descending aorta is right-sided.

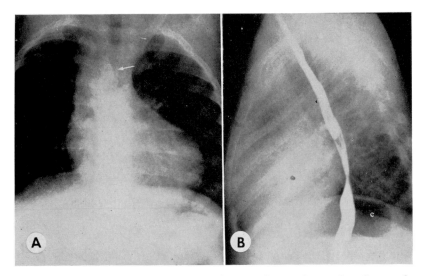

Figure 5-5. Case 2. Four-year-old child with tetralogy of Fallot, right aortic arch and mirror-image branching of the arch vessels. (*A*) The aortic arch indents the right side of the trachea (arrow). (*B*) Lateral view of the barium-filled esophagus showing no retroesophageal compression.

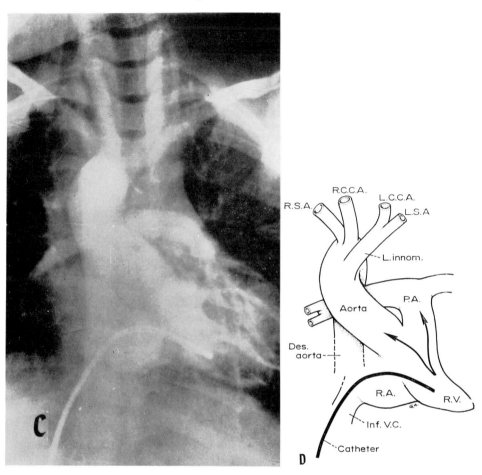

Figure 5-5. Case 2. (*C*) Selective right ventriculogram shows simultaneous opacification of the aorta and pulmonary artery. The first branch of the right arch is the left innominate artery followed by the right common carotid and right subclavian arteries. The aorta descends on the right. (*D*) Diagram of angiographic findings. (From W. H. Shuford, R. G. Sybers, and F. K. Edwards: The three types of right aortic arch. *Am J Roentgenol Radium Ther Nucl Med, 109*:67, 1970.)

Representative Cases

Case 3. Type 1 Right Aortic Arch. Six-year-old child with tetralogy of Fallot.

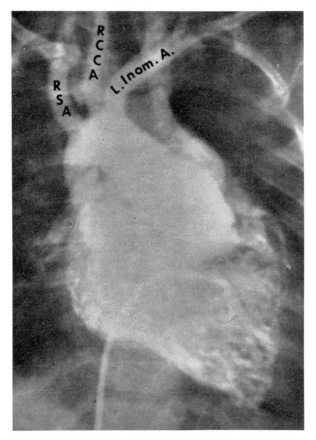

Figure 5-6. Case 3. Angiocardiogram in tetralogy of Fallot. The left innominate artery is the first branch off the right arch followed by the right common carotid and right subclavian arteries. The descending aorta is right-sided. (From W. H. Shuford, R. G. Sybers, and F. K. Edwards: The three types of right aortic arch. *Am J Roentgenol Radium Ther Nucl Med, 109:* 67, 1970.)

Case 4. Infant with persistent truncus arteriosus.

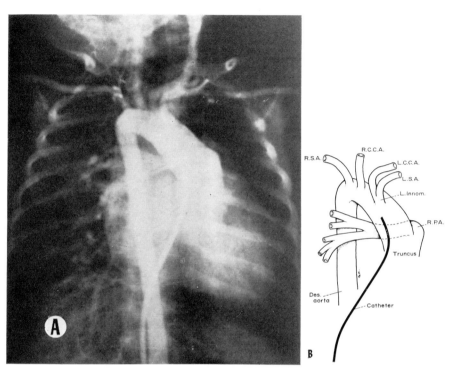

Figure 5-7. Case 4. Right aortic arch and truncus arteriosus. (*A*) Aortogram shows the truncus arteriosus. The first branch of the right arch is the left innominate artery which divides immediately into a left common carotid and a left subclavian artery. The second and third branches are the right common carotid and right subclavian arteries respectively. The right pulmonary artery arises directly from the proximal portion of the truncus arteriosus. Blood supply to the left lung is via systemic vessels from the descending aorta and arch. The aorta descends on the right side. (*B*) Drawing of aortogram.

Representative Cases

Case 5. Child with tetralogy of Fallot. (Courtesy of Squibb Hospital Division, E. R. Squibb & Sons, Inc. and Dr. Murray Baron.)

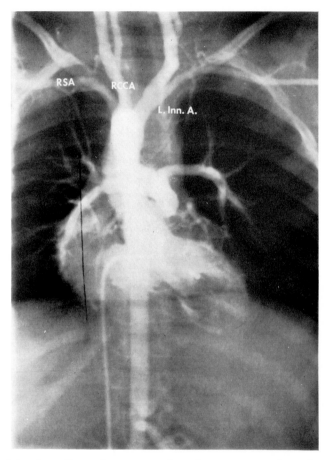

Figure 5-8. Case 5. Right aortic arch and mirror-image branching in tetralogy of Fallot. Right ventriculogram shows early filling of aorta and pulmonary artery. A left innominate artery is the first branch of the right arch. The right common carotid artery arises distal to the innominate artery and is followed by the right subclavian artery. (From Squibb X-Ray Atlas, Tetralogy of Fallot, May 1972, Figure 18, page 19.)

Type 2 Right Aortic Arch
(Mirror-image Branching—Rare Type)

Definition. In this type (Fig. 5-9) the right arch has three branches—a left innominate artery, a right common carotid artery and a right subclavian artery.[22, 25, 26] The left innominate artery courses anteriorly to the trachea and divides into a left common carotid artery and a left subclavian artery. The left ductus arteriosus extends from the upper descending aorta to the left pulmonary artery. An aortic diverticulum may be present at the aortic origin of the left ductus arteriosus.[28] A vascular ring is formed by the left ductus arteriosus.[28]

Clinical Significance. This anomaly is extremely rare.[4, 9, 14, 28] A complete vascular ring is present, and may be symptomatic.[28]

Development. Interruption of the embryonic left arch in the hypothetical double aortic arch between the left ductus arterio-

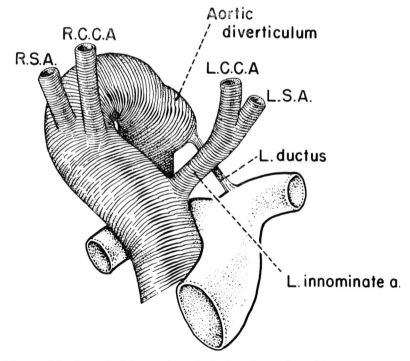

Figure 5-9. Type 2 right aortic arch (mirror-image branching—rare type). The first branch of the right arch is the left innominate artery. The distal right arch and aortic diverticulum produce a large retroesophageal defect.

sus and the left subclavian artery results in this malformation. The right ductus arteriosus usually disappears (Fig. 5-10).

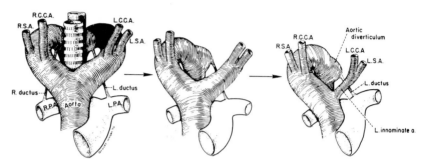

Figure 5-10. Development of Type 2 right aortic arch with mirror-image branching of the arch vessels and a left ductus arteriosus connecting the pulmonary artery to the descending aorta. There has been complete regression of the left arch in the hypothetical double aortic arch between the left subclavian artery and the left ductus in the area indicated in black. A vascular ring is present.

Chest Roentgenography. The frontal chest roentgenogram reveals a right aortic arch. Barium studies of the esophagus in this mirror-image type show posterior indentation produced by the vascular ring.[28]

Angiographic Features. Aortography demonstrates a right aortic arch giving rise to a left innominate artery, a right common carotid artery and a right subclavian artery in that order. An aortic diverticulum may be visible projecting from the left lateral wall of the upper descending aorta.[28]

Type 3 Right Aortic Arch
(Aberrant Left Subclavian Artery)

Definition. Four vessels originate from a right aortic arch in the following order—a left common carotid artery, a right common carotid artery, a right subclavian artery and an aberrant left subclavian artery. The left subclavian artery arises from the upper descending aorta as the fourth branch.[22, 25, 26] The aorta may descend either to the right or left of the spine.

Anatomic Variations. There are two anatomic variations. In one instance (Fig. 5-11), the aorta ascends to the right of the trachea and esophagus and the arch passes to the left behind the esophagus.[10, 17] The aorta usually descends on the left side of the spine. The left subclavian artery takes origin from a posterior diverticulum of the distal aortic arch. In this variation, the retroesophageal vascular component is large and represents principally the retroesophageal position of the aortic arch.[3] These cases have been referred to as right circumflex retroesophageal aortic arch.[15] A left ductus arteriosus extends from the aortic

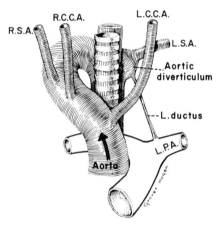

Figure 5-11. Type 3 right aortic arch (aberrant left subclavian artery). In this variation, the distal aortic arch is retroesophageal and the left ductus arteriosus connects to the aortic diverticulum.

diverticulum to the left pulmonary artery completing a vascular ring.[25]

In the other variation (Fig. 5-12), the aorta ascends sharply to the right of the trachea and esophagus, the arch continuing posteriorly to descend to the right of the spine.[17] The left subclavian artery arises from the descending aorta and courses obliquely behind the esophagus to reach the left arm.[17] In this variation, the retroesophageal vascular component is smaller and represents the left subclavian artery. The left ductus arteriosus connects the left subclavian artery to the left pulmonary artery completing a vascular ring.[7]

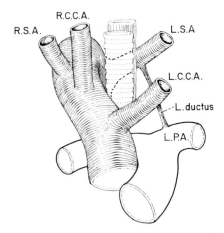

Figure 5-12. Type 3 right aortic arch (aberrant left subclavian artery). In this variation, the retroesophageal component is the left subclavian artery. The left ductus arteriosus connects to the left subclavian artery.

Incidence and Clinical Significance. Right aortic arch with an aberrant left subclavian artery is the most common type of right aortic arch.[3, 10, 22] The frequency of this occurrence is approximately ⅒ percent.[15] This type of right aortic arch is most often encountered as an incidental finding on routine chest roentgenogram or at necropsy.[5, 10, 26]

Right arch with an aberrant left subclavian artery forms a vascular ring encircling the trachea and esophagus. In a great majority of cases, however, the ring is loose and does not cause significant compression.[10, 26]

Only about 5% of patients with this anomaly have associated congenital heart disease. This type of arch branching is encountered in approximately 2% of patients with tetralogy of Fallot.[7]

Development. Right arch with an aberrant left subclavian artery results from interruption of the embryonic left arch in the hypothetical double aortic arch between the left subclavian artery and the left common carotid artery.[6, 8, 22] The proximal portion of the embryonic left arch forms the left common carotid artery which arises as the first branch of the aorta. The distal portion of the embryonic left arch persists as an aortic diverticulum giving rise to the left subclavian artery as the fourth branch of the right arch. The left ductus arteriosus is connected either to the aortic diverticulum (Fig. 5-13 or to the left subclavian artery (Fig. 5-14).

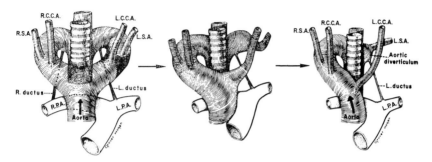

Figure 5-13. Development of Type 3 right aortic arch (aberrant left subclavian artery). There has been interruption of the left arch in the hypothetical double aortic arch between the left common carotid and the left subclavian arteries.

In this variation, the left subclavian artery arises from a posterior aortic diverticulum. The left ductus arteriosus extends between the left pulmonary artery and the diverticulum of the descending aorta. The retroesophageal component is the posterior right aortic arch.

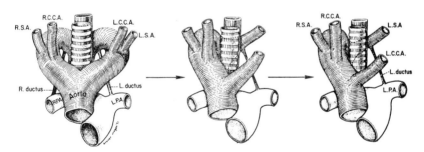

Figure 5-14. Development of Type 3 right aortic arch (aberrant left subclavian artery). There has been interruption of the left arch in the hypothetical double aortic arch between the left common carotid artery and the left subclavian artery.

In this variation, the left subclavian artery arises from the distal arch. The left ductus arteriosus extends between the left pulmonary artery and the left subclavian artery. The retroesophageal component is the left subclavian artery.

Chest Roentgenography. On the frontal view, the right aortic arch indents the right side of the trachea.[3, 10] The right aortic arch is frequently higher than the position of the normal left arch.[5] The descending aorta is either to the right or left of the midline. A convex soft tissue shadow, representing the persistent distal left embryonic arch (posterior aortic diverticulum) is often visible along the left upper mediastinal border.[18, 22] Most often in patients with this arch anomaly, the heart has a normal appearance.[3, 15]

On the lateral chest roentgenogram, frequentlyy a large rounded superior mediastinal mass is visible displacing the trachea anteriorly. This soft tissue shadow represents either the retroesophageal component of the right arch or the aortic diverticulum.[22]

Barium examination of the esophagus in the frontal projection, in addition to a vascular impression on the right side, may show an oblique filling defect extending upward from right to left just below the aortic arch.[3] Lateral studies of the esophagus often are diagnostic, showing a large retroesophageal vascular defect produced by the right arch or the junction of the posterior aortic diverticulum and the left subclavian artery.[10]

Angiographic Features. The ascending aorta arises to the right of the trachea and esophagus. The first branch of the right arch is the left common carotid artery followed by the right common carotid artery, right subclavian artery, and the left subclavian artery.[22] Often, an aortic diverticulum is visible at the origin of the left subclavian artery.[3, 22] The descending aorta may be either on the right or left side of the spine.[17]

On rare occasions, the proximal portion of the aberrant left subclavian artery may be stenotic. Angiograms will demonstrate the stenotic zone (Case 11, Figs. 5-20, 5-21). When the stenosis is severe, or when the aberrant left subclavian artery is atretic, the left subclavian artery does not opacify from the aorta but receives blood by collateral flow through the left vertebral artery. Under these circumstances, the angiographic findings resemble those of the right aortic arch with isolation of the left subclavian artery. (See RIGHT AORTIC ARCH WITH ISOLATION OF THE LEFT SUBCLAVIAN ARTERY—DIFFERENTIAL DIAGNOSIS in Chapter 5).

Representative Cases

Case 6. Asymptomatic adult patient.

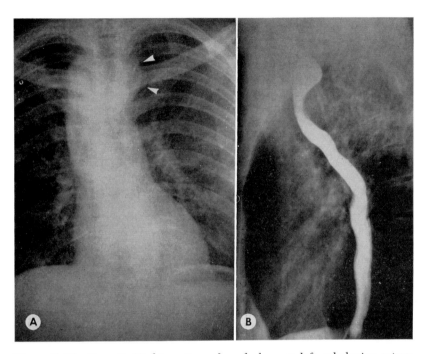

Figure 5-15. Case 6. Right aortic arch and aberrant left subclavian artery. (A) The ascending aorta arches far to the right. An aortic diverticulum projects as a soft tissue density to the left of the spine (arrows). The descending aorta is on the left. (B) Lateral esophagogram. A large retroesophageal vascular impression is visible. (From W. H. Shuford, R. G. Sybers, and F. K. Edwards: The three types of right aortic arch. *Am J Roentgenol Radium Ther Nucl Med, 109:67,* 1970.)

Case 7. A fifty-two-year-old man with history of chronic alcoholism and malnutrition, hospitalized with anemia and hepatomegaly. No evidence of heart disease.

Blood pressure 138/80 mm Hg in both arms. The examination of the heart was negative.

Chest roentgenogram showed a questionable mass in the superior mediastinum. Aortography (Fig. 5-16) revealed a right aortic arch with the left common carotid, right common carotid and right subclavian arteries arising from the arch in that order. On the left there was a diverticulum-like outpouching of the aorta from which arose the left subclavian artery.

Representative Cases

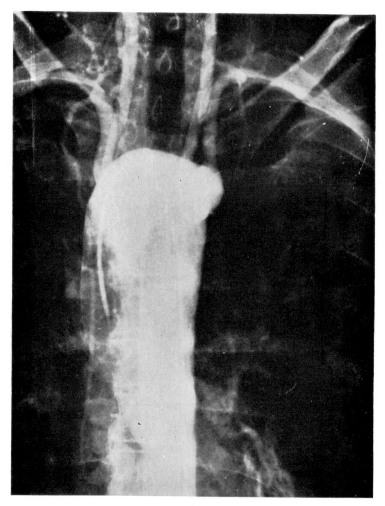

Figure 5-16. (A)

Figure 5-16. Case 7. Right aortic arch and aberrant left subclavian artery.
(A) The left subclavian artery originates from a diverticulum-like structure
of the aorta. (B) Right posterior oblique projection. Left common carotid
artery arises as first branch off the arch, followed by right common carotid,
right subclavian and left subclavian arteries. (C) Diagram of B. (From
W. H. Shuford, R. G. Sybers, and F. K. Edwards: The three types of right
aortic arch. *Am J Roentgenol Radium Ther Nucl Med, 109*:67, 1970.)

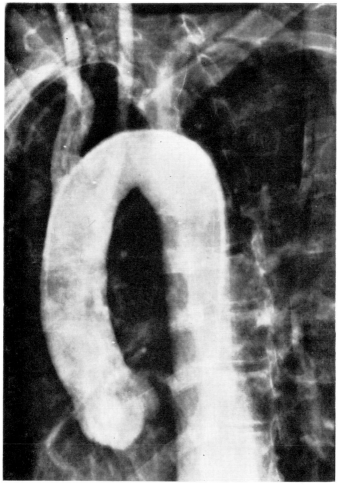

Figure 5-16. (B)

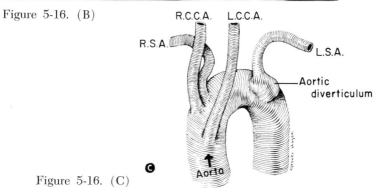

Figure 5-16. (C)

Representative Cases

Case 8. Child with tetralogy of Fallot.

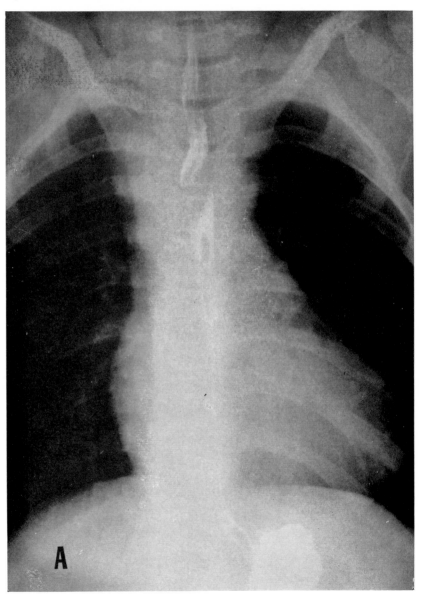

Figure 5-17. Case 8. Tetralogy of Fallot with right aortic arch and aberrant left subclavian artery. (A) Chest roentgenogram shows moderate cardiomegaly. The pulmonary artery segment is small. The shadow of the descending aorta is to the right of the spine. The barium-filled esophagus shows an oblique filling defect extending upward from right to left.

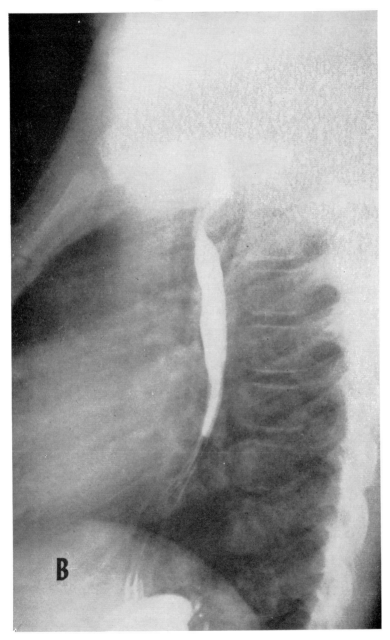

Figure 5-17. Case 8. Tetralogy of Fallot with right aortic arch and aberrant left subclavian artery. Lateral esophagogram (*B*) shows a prominent retroesophageal vascular impression at the level of the aortic arch.

Representative Cases

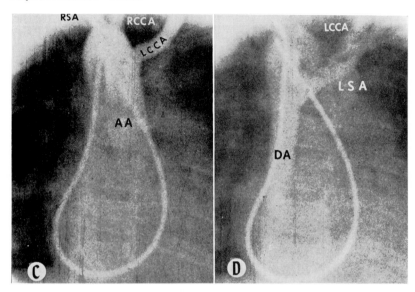

Figure 5-17. Case 8. Tetralogy of Fallot with right aortic arch and aberrant left subclavian artery. Cineaortograms (*C* & *D*). The catheter has passed from the right ventricle through a ventricular septal defect into the ascending aorta. There is a right aortic arch. The left common carotid artery is the first branch, followed by the right common carotid artery, right subclavian artery and left subclavian artery. The aberrant left subclavian artery arises from the upper descending aorta and compresses the posterior wall of the esophagus. RSA = right subclavian artery, RCCA = right common carotid artery, LCCA = left common carotid artery, AA = ascending aorta, DA = descending aorta, LSA = left subclavian artery.

Case 9. A five-year-old child with a ventricular septal defect and associated right aortic arch. (Figure 5-18 *A-D.*) (From J. E. Edwards, L. S. Carey, H. N. Neufeld, and R. G. Lester: *Congenital Heart Disease.* Philadelphia, Saunders, 1965, vol. 1, p. 171.)

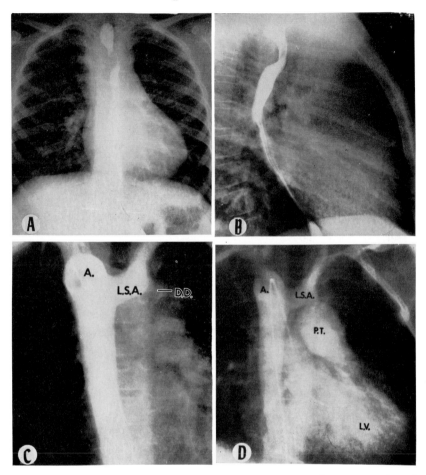

Figure 5-18. Case 9. Ventricular septal defect with right aortic arch and aberrant left subclavian artery. (*A & B*) Frontal and lateral esophagograms show deformity of the upper portion of the barium-filled esophagus produced by the retroesophageal course of the aberrant left subclavian artery. Slight cardiomegaly. (*C*) Selective retrograde aortogram shows right aortic arch, right-sided descending aorta and the left subclavian artery (LSA) arising as the fourth branch of the upper descending aorta. A small outpouching (DD) of the left subclavian artery represents the systemic remnant of the ligamentum arteriosum which connects the left subclavian artery to the left pulmonary artery. (*D*) Selective left ventriculogram. There is simultaneous opacification of the aorta and pulmonary trunk following injection of contrast material into the left ventricle. The pulmonary artery fills via a left-to-right shunt through a ventricular septal defect.

Representative Cases

Case 10.   Child with tetralogy of Fallot. (Fig. 5-19 *A* & *B*). (Courtesy of Squibb Hospital Division, E. R. Squibb & Sons, Inc. and Dr. Murray Baron.)

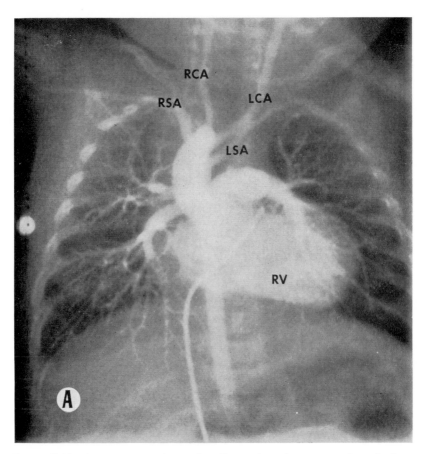

Figure 5-19. Case 10. Tetralogy of Fallot with right aortic arch and aberrant left subclavian artery. (*A*) Selective right ventriculogram. The left subclavian artery arises as the fourth branch of the right aortic arch. The left common carotid artery is the first branch, followed by the right common carotid and right subclavian artery. The descending aorta is right-sided. Simultaneous opacification of aorta and pulmonary artery from right ventricle.

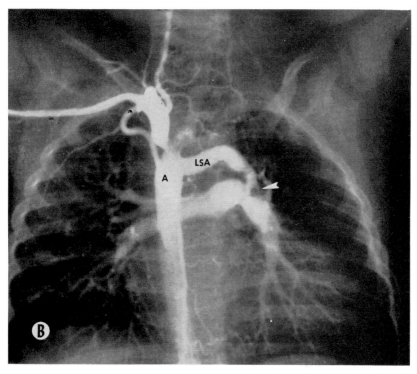

Figure 15-19. Case 10. Tetralogy of Fallot with right aortic arch and aberrant left subclavian artery. Post-Blalock anastomosis. Selective injection of contrast material into descending aorta. The left subclavian artery delivers blood to the pulmonary artery through a patent anastomosis (arrow). (From Squibb X-Ray Atlas, Tetralogy of Fallot, May 1972, Figures 19 and 20, p. 20.)

Representative Cases

Case 11. *Right aortic arch with coarctation of proximal portion of aber-*
rant left subclavian artery producing tracheoesophageal constriction.
This seven-week-old infant was admitted with a history of rapid respirations, cough and an episode of cyanosis, apnea and loss of con-
sciousness.

Pulse rate was 140 per minute. Blood pressure was 90 mm Hg
in the right arm and left leg. A grade III systolic murmur was audible at the left sternal border. Cardiac catheterization showed a ventricular septal defect. Chest films revealed cardiac enlargement and
increased pulmonary blood flow. On barium swallow studies, there
was an oblique pressure defect running upward from right to left
behind the esophagus.

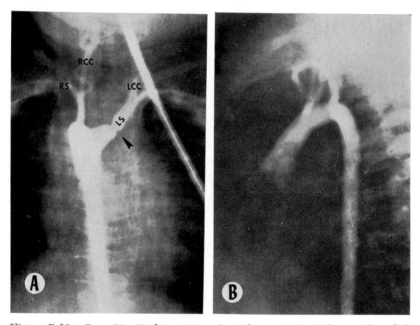

Figure 5-20. Case 11. Right aortic arch with coarctation of anomalous left
subclavian artery and vascular ring. Frontal (*A*) and lateral (*B*) aortograms
show right-sided aortic arch and descending aorta. There is stenosis (arrow)
of the proximal portion of the left subclavian artery which arises as the last
branch of the right arch. (From T. E. Keats, and J. M. Martt: Tracheoesophageal constriction produced by an unusual combination of anomalies
of the great vessels. *Am Heart J, 63:265, 1962.*)

Retrograde aortography (Fig. 5-20 *A* & *B*) showed a right aortic arch with a right descending aorta. The first vessel off the arch was the left common carotid artery, followed by the right common carotid artery, then the right subclavian artery, and lastly the left subclavian artery which was directed behind the esophagus. The proximal portion of the aberrant left subclavian artery was stenosed. Figure 5-21 is a diagrammatic representation of the vascular anomaly. The left subclavian artery and the left ligamentum arteriosum were transected to relieve the tracheoesophageal obstruction.

Postmortem examination revealed a large ventricular septal defect, right-sided aortic arch, and anomalous origin of the left subclavian artery. (Courtesy of Dr. Theodore E. Keats.)

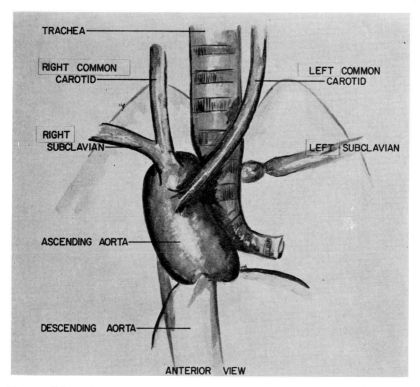

Figure 5-21. Case 11. Diagrammatic representation of the vascular anomaly. (From T. E. Keats, and J. M. Martt: Tracheoesophageal constriction produced by an unusual combination of anomalies of the great vessels. *Am Heart J, 63*:265, 1962.)

Representative Cases

Case 12. Right aortic arch with aberrant left subclavian artery producing a vascular ring. This ten-month-old boy suffered with symptoms of tracheal and esophageal obstruction since birth. Chest film showed the aortic arch to the right of the trachea and slightly more cephalad than the normal left arch. Barium swallow (Fig. 5-22 A & B) revealed a large retroesophageal concavity with compression defects on both sides of the esophagus.

Aortography (Fig. 5-22 C & D) confirmed the presence of a right aortic arch with the left common carotid artery arising as the first branch, followed by the right common carotid and right subclavian arteries. The left subclavian artery originated as the last branch of the distal arch.

At operation, a tight vascular ring was present, formed by the pulmonary artery and ascending aorta anteriorly, the aortic arch on the right, the aortic arch and upper descending aorta posteriorly, and the left dorsal aortic root and the left ductus arteriosus on the left. The ductus arteriosus and the left subclavain artery were divided. The patient was asymptomatic three months after operation. (Courtesy of Dr. Owings W. Kincaid.)

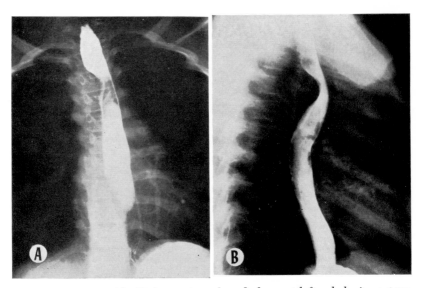

Figure 5-22. Case 12. Right aortic arch and aberrant left subclavian artery. Frontal (A) and lateral (B) esophagograms show retroesophageal and bilateral compression defects of the esophagus.

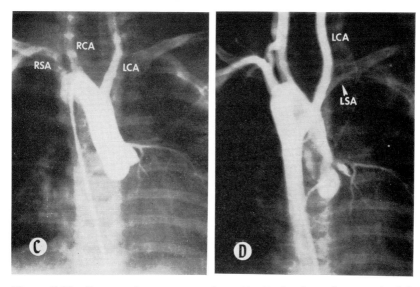

Figure 5-22. Retrograde aortogram. Case 12. Early phase showing the left common carotid artery as the first branch of the proximal arch. (*D*) Later film demonstrates the right common carotid artery and the right subclavian artery to arise distal to the left carotid artery. There is faint opacification of the left subclavian artery (arrow) which originates as the fourth branch from a conical aortic diverticulum. (From A. R. Wychulis, O. W. Kincaid, W. H. Weidman, and G. K. Danielson: Congenital vascular ring: surgical considerations and results of operation. *Mayo Clin Proc, 46*:182, 1971.)

Type 4 Right Aortic Arch
(Aberrant Left Innominate Artery)

Definition. In this type of right arch (Fig. 5-23), the left innominate artery arises as the third branch from the distal right arch, passing behind the esophagus to give origin to the left common carotid and left subclavian arteries.[13] A vascular ring is present, formed by the right arch, posteriorly by the retroesophageal left innominate artery, and on the left by the left ductus arteriosus.[13]

Incidence and Clinical Significance. Only a few well-documented cases have been reported.[13] It may form a symptomatic vascular ring.

Development. This anomaly results from interruption of the

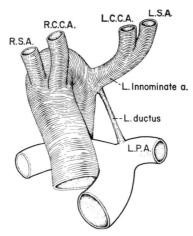

Figure 5-23. Type 4 aortic arch (aberrant left innominate artery). The right common carotid artery is the first branch followed by the right sub-clavian artery and the left innominate artery. A vascular ring is present.

embryonic left arch in the hypothetical double aortic arch be-tween the ascending aorta and the left common carotid artery. The right ductus arteriosus disappears (Fig. 5-24).[6, 8]

Chest Roentgenography. The frontal chest x-ray shows a right aortic arch. Barium studies reveal a posterior compression defect on the esophagus at the level of the aortic arch.[13]

Angiographic Features. The aorta arches to the right of the trachea. The first branch of the right arch is the right common carotid artery, followed by the right subclavian artery and the

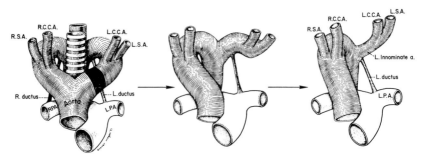

Figure 5-24. Development of Type 4 right aortic arch (aberrant left in-nominate artery). There has been interruption of the left embryonic arch in the hypothetical double aortic arch (area in black) between the ascend-ing aorta and left common carotid artery.

left innominate artery arises as the third branch from the upper descending aorta.[13]

Representative Case

Case 13. This nineteen-year-old man was hospitalized because of a heart murmur and exertional dyspnea. Past history reveals hospitalization during the first year of life with a diagnosis of mucoviscidosis and aspiration pneumonia. There had been difficulty with feeding associated with cough and dyspnea.

Physical examination revealed the blood pressure in all extremities to be within normal limits. A loud diamond-shaped systolic murmur was heard at the upper left sternal border.

Chest roentgenograms with barium (Fig. 5-25 A & B) revealed a right aortic arch with a rather large retroesophageal indentation of the opacified esophagus.

Left heart catheterization confirmed the presence of valvular aortic stenosis. Thoracic aortography (Fig. 5-26) showed the pres-

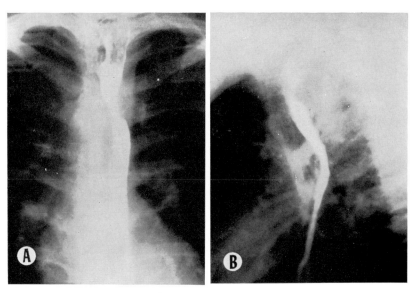

Figure 5-25. Case 13. Right aortic arch with an aberrant retroesophageal innominate artery. Frontal chest roentgenogram with barium (A) demonstrates normal-appearing heart and lungs. The right aortic arch displaces the esophagus to the left. (B) Lateral view shows posterior indentation of the esophagus suggestive of a retroesophageal vessel. (From J. H. Grollman, H. S. Henderson, and R. J. Hall: Right aortic arch with aberrant retroesophageal innominate artery: angiographic diagnosis. (*Radiology,* 90:782, 1968.)

Representative Cases

ence of a right aortic arch from which a retroesophageal innominate artery arose as the last vessel. Surgery was not recommended. (Courtesy of Dr. Julius H. Grollman, Jr.)

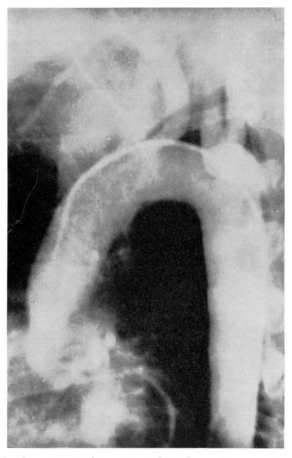

Figure 5-26. Case 13. Right aortic arch with an aberrant retroesophageal innominate artery. Aortogram (right posterior oblique projection). The left innominate artery is the last branch off the arch and gives rise to the left subclavian and left common carotid arteries. The right common carotid artery and the right subclavian artery are the first two branches of the right arch. (From J. H. Grollman, H. S. Henderson, and R. J. Hall: Right aortic arch with aberrant retroesophageal innominate artery:angiographic diagnosis. *Radiology*, 90:782, 1968.)

Type 5 Right Aortic Arch
(Isolation of the Left Subclavian Artery)

Definition. In this malformation (Fig. 5-27), the left common carotid artery, the right common carotid and right subclavian arteries arise independently from the aortic arch in that order.[2] The left subclavian artery no longer has a connection with the aorta, but is connected to the left pulmonary artery by way of a left ductus arteriosus.[23, 25] The right arch is anterior to the trachea and esophagus, and a vascular ring is not present.[23]

Incidence and Clinical Significance. Right aortic arch with isolation of the left subclavian artery is an uncommon congenital anomaly. This anomaly is frequently associated with cyanotic congenital heart disease, especially tetralogy of Fallot.[12, 25] Some patients with this aortic arch malformation have not had heart disease.[20, 23] In these cases, the clinical symptoms have resulted from the associated subclavian steal syndrome, either in the form

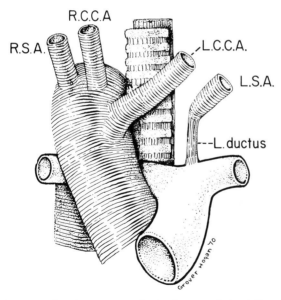

Figure 5-27. Type 5 right aortic arch (isolation of the left subclavian artery). The left subclavian artery is connected to the left pulmonary artery by the left ductus arteriosus.

of cerebral symptoms or difference in blood pressure and pulse between the two arms.[20, 23]

Development. This malformation can be explained by interruption of the embryonic left arch in the hypothetical double aortic arch at two levels: one between the left common carotid and left subclavian arteries, and the other distal to the origin of the left subclavian artery (Fig. 5-28).[2, 23] The proximal portion of the embryonic left arch becomes the left common carotid artery and arises as the first branch of the right arch to be followed by the right common carotid and right subclavian arteries.

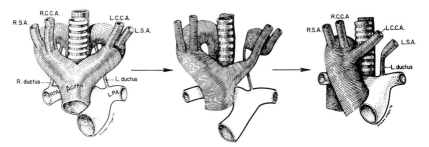

Figure 5-28. Development of Type 5 right aortic arch (isolation of the left subclavian artery). Areas in black indicate sites of interruption in embryonic left arch in the hypothetical double aortic arch.

There may be persistence of the most distal portion of the embryonic left arch. In this event, a diverticulum-like structure is present along the inner aspect of the distal right arch (Fig. 5-29). The development of this aortic diverticulum is shown in Figure 5-30.

This aortic diverticulum does not represent the attachment of the left ductus arteriosus, as the left ductus connects to the left subclavian artery rather than to the descending aorta.

Chest Roentgenography. The frontal chest x-ray shows the aortic knob and descending aorta to be on the right side.[20, 23] Cardiac enlargement and decreased pulmonary vasculature may be present in patients with tetralogy of Fallot.

The esophagogram shows displacement of the esophagus to the left at the level of the aortic arch. However, there is no pos-

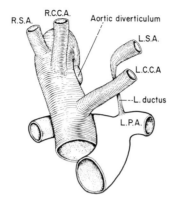

Figure 5-29. Right aortic arch and isolation of the left subclavian artery with an aortic diverticulum of the descending aorta.

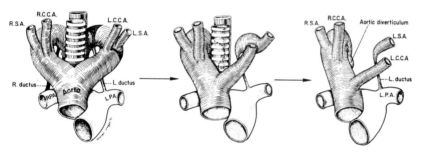

Figure 5-30. Development of right aortic arch and isolation of the left subclavian artery with an aortic diverticulum of the distal arch. The most posterior portion of the left embryonic arch persists forming a diverticulum of the distal right arch. Areas in black indicate sites of interruption in embryonic left arch in the hypothetical double aortic arch.

terior defect on the barium-filled esophagus, as a vascular ring is not present.[23, 24]

Angiographic Features. The ascending aorta passes upward in a straight line, to the right of the trachea and esophagus, and descends on the right of the spine. The left common carotid artery opacifies as the first branch of the aortic arch, and is followed by the right common carotid and right subclavian arteries in that order. The left subclavian artery does not opacify from the arch, but receives blood thorough collateral circulation.[20, 23, 24]

Representative Cases

Case 14. This twenty-three-year-old soldier at age seven was found to have a difference in blood pressure between the two arms. Later he noticed that his left arm tired more easily. There were no symptoms to suggest congenital heart disease or cerebral or vertebrobasilar insufficiency.

Blood pressure in the right arm was 118/50 mm Hg, and 80/56 mm Hg in the left arm. The left radial and antecubital pulses were markedly diminished when the extremity was dependent and disappeared when the left arm was raised above the shoulder. Examination of the heart was negative.

Chest x-ray revealed a right aortic arch (Fig. 5-31 A & B). The heart and pulmonary vasculature were normal. Esophagograms in both anterior oblique positions showed no abnormal defect on the esophagus. (Fig. 5-31 C & D).

Percutaneous catheter aortography with injection of opaque material into the ascending aorta showed a right aortic arch. The left common carotid artery originated as the first branch and was followed by the right common carotid and right subclavian arteries. The left subclavian artery did not opacify from the arch. The descending aorta was on the right (Fig. 5-32). Figure 5-33 A shows a selective injection of the left common carotid artery. Approximately two seconds following the injection (Fig. 5-33 B & C), the left subclavian artery was opacified by collateral channels from the occipital branch of the left external carotid artery to branches of the thyrocervical and costocervical trunks of the left subclavian artery. In addition, there was abnormal opacification of the left vertebral artery by way of muscular branches of the occipital artery with retrograde flow down the vertebral artery, contributing blood to the left subclavian vessel. The left inferior thyroid artery of the thyrocervical trunk received blood directly from the left superior thyroid branch of the external carotid artery.

A second injection of the left comomn carotid artery revealed no blood reaching the left vertebral artery through the circle of Willis.

Percutaneous catheterization of the left brachial artery was then performed. Upon advancement, the catheter met resistance in the first or thoracic portion of the left subclavian artery. Hand injection of contrast material showed this segment of the left subclavian artery to end blindly with no visible connection with either the aortic arch or with the left pulmonary artery. There was filling of the vertebral, costocervical and thyrocervical trunks of the left subclavian artery Fig. 5-34 A & B).

Figure 5-35 shows a diagram of possible routes of collateral flow in the presence of an occlusion or absence of the first portion of the left subclavian artery.

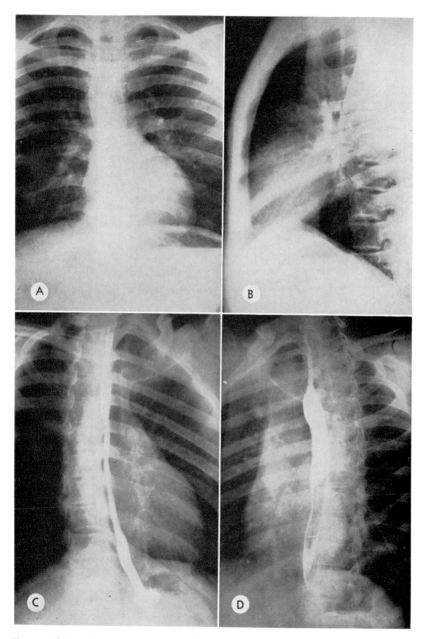

Figure 5-31. Case 14. (*A* and *B*) Right aortic arch and isolation of the left subclavian artery. The heart is not enlarged. In the lateral view the trachea shows no posterior compression. (*C* and *D*) Right and left anterior oblique esophagograms. There is no defect on the posterior aspect of the esophagus. (From W. H. Shuford, R. G. Sybers, and R. C. Schlant: Right aortic arch with isolation of the left subclavian artery. *Am J Roentgenol Radium Ther Nucl Med, 109:*75, 1970.)

Representative Cases

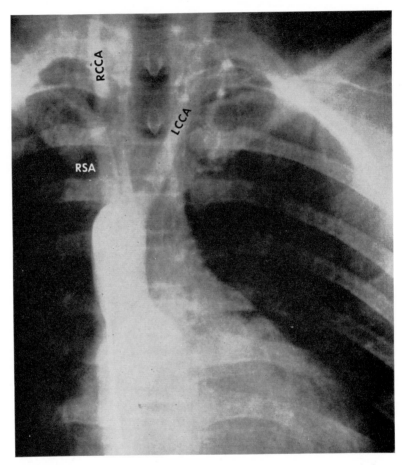

Figure 5-32. Case 14. Right aortic arch and isolation of the left subclavian artery. The descending aorta is on the right. There is opacification of the left common carotid, right common carotid and right subclavian arteries only from the arch. (From W. H. Shuford, R. G. Sybers, and R. C. Schlant: Right aortic arch with isolation of the left subclavian artery. *Am J Roentgenol Radium Ther Nucl Med, 109*:75, 1970.)

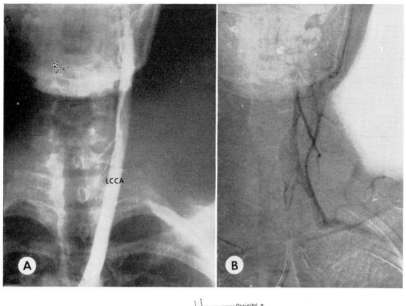

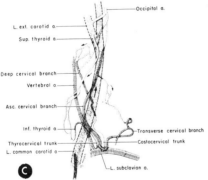

Figure 5-33. Case 14. (*A*) Selective injection of the left common carotid artery. (*B*) Subtraction arteriogram two seconds following injection. The left external carotid artery supplies the vertebral artery, the inferior thyroid artery, the thyrocervical and costocervical trunks with retrograde flow opacifying the left subclavian artery distal to the vertebral origin. The thoracic portion of the left subclavian artery is not opacified. (*C*) Composite drawing of *A* and *B*. (From W. H. Shuford, R. G. Sybers, and R. C. Schlant: Right aortic arch with isolation of the left subclavian artery. *Am J Roentgenol Radium Ther Nucl Med, 109:75, 1970.*)

Representative Cases

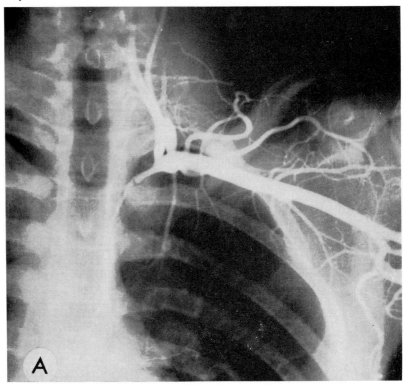

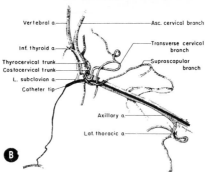

Figure 5-34. Case 14. (*A*) Retrograde injection of the left subclavian artery. Catheter tip is in the first portion of the left subclavian artery. (*B*) Drawing of *A*. No connection of the left subclavian artery with the aortic arch or left pulmonary artery can be seen. (From W. H. Shuford, R. G. Sybers, and R. C. Schlant: Right aortic arch with isolation of the left subclavian artery. *Am J Roentgenol Radium Ther Nucl Med, 109:75*, 1970.)

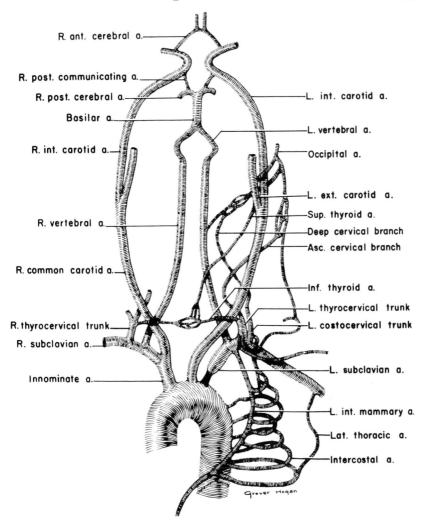

Figure 5-35. Case 14. Diagram of collateral circulation in the presence of occlusion or absence of the first portion of the left subclavian artery. (From W. H. Shuford, R. G. Sybers, and R. G. Schlant: Subclavian steal syndrome in right aortic arch with isolation of the left subclavian artery. *Am Heart J, 82*:98, 1971.)

Representative Cases

Case 15. This thirty-four-year-old man was admitted with the diagnosis of chronic schizophrenia. Except for mental illness, he was of good health. Apparently, he experienced no difficulty with the use of his left arm.

On examination, the patient was in good physical condition. Pulse

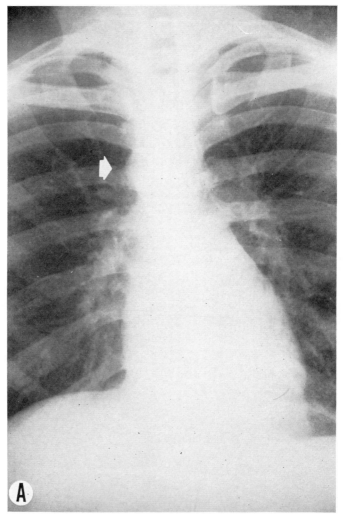

Figure 5-36. Case 15. (A) Right aortic arch (arrow) with isolation of the left subclavian artery. The heart has a normal configuration with no abnormality of the pulmonary vasculature.

rate and blood pressure were normal in the right arm and were unobtainable in the left arm. The examination of the heart revealed no abnormal findings.

Chest roentgenograms and a barium swallow examination showed a right aortic arch and a heart of normal size. The pulmonary artery segment and pulmonary vasculature were unremarkable. There was no defect visible on the posterior esophageal wall. (Fig. 5-36 A & B).

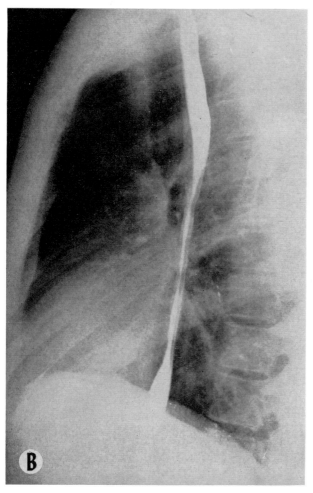

Figure 5-36 B. Case 15. The barium-filled esophagus shows no retroesophageal compression. (From W. H. Shuford, R. G. Sybers, and R. C. Schlant: Right aortic arch with isolation of the left subclavian artery. *Am J Roentgenol Radium Ther Nucl Med, 109*:75, 1970.)

Representative Cases

Because of the absent pulse in the left arm, percutaneous catheter aortography was performed. Injection of contrast material into the ascending aorta showed a right arch with filling of the left common carotid, right common carotid and right subclavian arteries in that order. The left subclavian artery did not opacify from the aorta (Fig. 5-37 *A*). Serial studies at two to three seconds after injection revealed faint opacification of a small, tortuous left subclavian artery which filled by retrograde flow down the left vertebral artery (Fig. 5-37 *B* & *C*). The descending aorta was on the right. On the lateral aortogram, a diverticulum-like structure was present at the junction of the origin of the descending aorta (Fig. 5-38).

The developmental basis for this aortic diverticulum is illustrated in Figure 5-30.

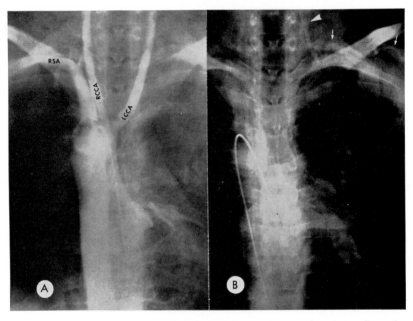

Figure 5-37. Case 15. (*A*) Aortogram showing the aortic arch on the right, a right-sided descending aorta, and the left common carotid, right common carotid and right subclavian arteries arising from the arch in that order. There is no opacification of the left subclavian artery from the arch. (*B*) Two seconds after injection reversed flow in the left vertebral artery (upper arrow) opacifies the left subclavian artery distal to the vertebral origin (lower arrows).

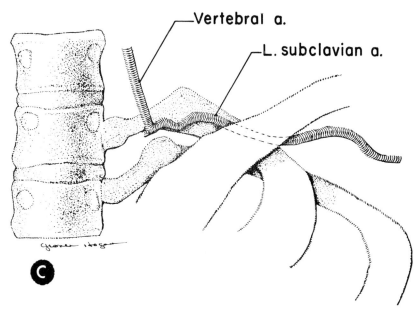

Figure 5-37 C. Case 15. Diagram of arteriogram in *B*. (From W. H. Shuford, R. G. Sybers, and R. C. Schlant: Right aortic arch with isolation of the left subclavian artery. *Am J Roentgenol Radium Ther Nucl Med,* *109*:75, 1970.)

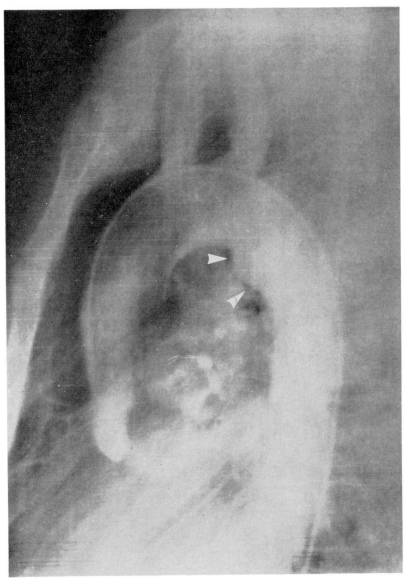

Figure 5-38. Case 15. Right aortic arch with isolation of the left sub-clavian artery. Lateral aortogram showing diverticulum-like structure (arrows) at the junction of the arch and descending aorta. In this patient this structure represents persistence of a portion of the most distal embryonic left arch. It is not the so-called "ductus diverticulum" as the left ductus arteriosus connects to the left subclavian artery rather than to the descending aorta. The development of this aortic diverticulum is shown in Figure 5-30. (From W. H. Shuford, R. G. Sybers, and R. C. Schlant: Right aortic arch with isolation of the left subclavian artery. *Am J Roentgenol Radium Ther Nucl Med,* 109:75, 1970.)

DIFFERENTIAL DIAGNOSIS OF RIGHT AORTIC ARCH WITH ISOLATION OF THE LEFT SUBCLAVIAN ARTERY

In the differential diagnosis of right aortic arch with isolation of the left subclavian artery, one other condition must be given consideration, namely right aortic arch and aberrant left subclavian artery with atresia or severe stenosis of the left subclavian artery.

In this anomaly (Fig. 5-39), the proximal portion of the left subclavian artery is atretic or tightly stenotic.[27] The left subclavian artery may arise from a diverticulum of the descending aorta which represents persistence of the embryonic left dorsal aortic root.[1] A left ductus arteriosus completes the left side of the vascular ring.[1]

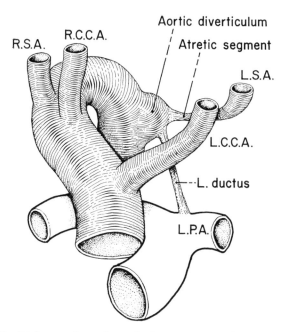

Figure 5-39. Right aortic arch and aberrant left subclavian artery with partial atresia of the left subclavian artery. The angiographic findings in this anomaly are identical to right aortic arch and isolation of the left subclavian artery.

The development of this malformation is shown in Figure 5-40 and results from complete interruption of the embryonic left arch in the hypothetical double aortic arch between the left common carotid artery and the left subclavian artery, with partial regression of the embryonic left arch between the left ductus and left subclavian artery.

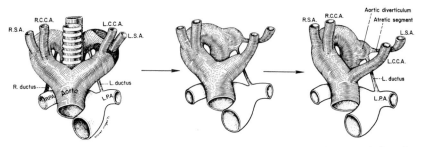

Figure 5-40. Development of the right aortic arch and aberrant left subclavian artery with partial atresia of the left subclavian artery. There has been complete regression of the left arch in the hypothetical double aortic arch between the left common carotid and left subclavian artery (black area) and partial regression of the left arch distal to the left subclavian artery (shaded area).

Only a few cases of this arch anomaly have been diagnosed during life. [1, 11, 16, 19, 27] This arch malformation has the same angiographic features as right aortic arch with isolation of the left subclavian artery.[1, 11, 27] However, a vascular ring is present in this arch malformation, and the presence of a retroesophageal indentation on the lateral esophagogram would differentiate right aortic arch with an atretic aberrant left subclavian artery from right aortic arch and isolation of the left subclavian artery.[23]

Representative Case

Case 16. Right Aortic Arch and Aberrant Left Subclavian Artery with Atresia of the Proximal Portion of the Left Subclavian Artery. This two-month-old female infant was hospitalized with severe congestive heart failure and respiratory distress.

Physical examination showed a small cyanotic infant in severe respiratory distress. A holosystolic murmur was heard along the left sternal border. The left brachial and radial arterial pulses were diminished.

Chest roentgenograms (Fig. 5-41 A & B) showed prominent pulmonary vasculature, cardiomegaly with left atrial enlargement and pulmonary infiltrations. A right aortic arch was present. The lateral view showed a concave impression in the posterior wall of the esophagus at the level of the aortic arch.

Cardiac catheterization demonstrated a large left-to-right shunt at the ventricular level. Left ventriculography (Fig. 5-42 A, B, C) revealed a ventricular septal defect, a right aortic arch and a prominent diverticulum of the distal arch. The left subclavian artery did not opacify from the aorta, but filled by way of collateral flow from left vertebral artery. Both carotid arteries and the right subclavian artery filled from the arch. Postmortem examination of the heart revealed a large ventricular septal defect with overriding aorta, partial anomalous venous connection of the right upper lobe veins, a right aortic arch with an aortic diverticulum at the junction of the upper

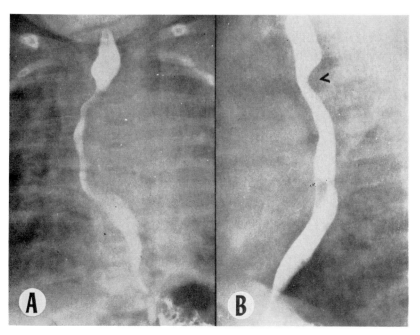

Figure 5-41. Case 16. Right aortic arch with atresia of the aberrant left subclavian artery. (A) A right aortic arch indents the right side of the esophagus. There is increased pulmonary vasculature. Lateral esophagogram (B) shows a large concave retroesophageal defect (arrow). From B. E. Victorica, L. H. S. Van Mierop, and L. P. Elliott: Right aortic arch associated with contralateral congenital subclavian steal syndrome. *Am J Roentgenol Radium Ther Nucl Med,* 108:582, 1970.)

Representative Cases

and descending aorta and distal arch, and a left posterior ductus arteriosus. The left subclavian artery originated from the aortic diverticulum, but its proximal portion was atretic. (Courtesy of Dr. Larry P. Elliott.)

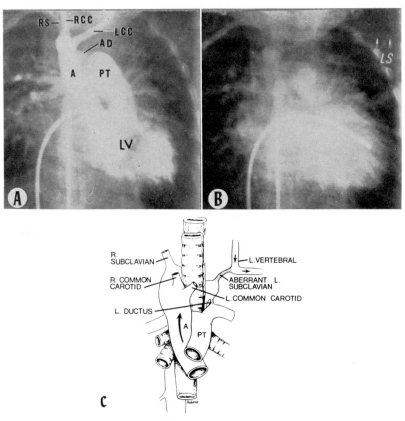

Figure 5-42. Case 16. Right aortic arch with atresia of the aberrant left subclavian artery. (A) Left ventriculogram shows a large ventricular septal defect, a right aortic arch and an aortic diverticulum behind the esophagus. Both carotid arteries and the right subclavian artery arise from the aorta. (B) The left subclavian artery opacifies late (arrows) via the left vertebral artery, with no visible connection to the aorta. (C) Schematic drawing of the arch anomaly. (From B. E. Victorica, L. H. S. Mierop, and L. R. Elliott: Right aortic arch associated with contralateral congenital subclavian steal syndrome. *Am J Roentgenol Radium Ther Nucl Med, 108:*582, 1970.)

Theoretically, two other congenital anomalies may show angiographic findings similar to those of right aortic arch with isolation of the left subclavian artery.

1. Double aortic arch with atresia in the left arch between the left common carotid and left subclavian arteries, and a second area of atresia in the left arch between the origin of the left subclavian artery and the descending aorta.
2. Right aortic arch with mirror-image branching and atresia between the left common carotid artery and the left subclavian artery.

However, both of these arch anomalies remain hypothetical possibilities, as there are no reported examples of these malformations.[25]

REFERENCES

1. Antia, A. U., and Ottesen, O. E.: Collateral circulation in subclavian stenosis or atresia. *Am J Cardiol, 18*:599, 1966.
2. Barger, J. D.; Bregman, E. H., and Edwards, J. E.: Bilateral ductus arteriosus with right aortic arch and right-sided descending aorta. *Am J Roentgenol Radium Ther Nucl Med, 76*:758, 1956.
3. Baron, M. G.: Right aortic arch. *Circulation, 44*:1137, 1971.
4. Baronfsky, I. D.; Kreel, I.; Steinfeld, L., and Grishman, A.: Vascular ring in infancy. *NY State J Med, 60*:1246, 1960.
5. Bedford, D. E., and Parkinson, J.: Right-sided aortic arch. *Br J Radiol, 108*:776, 1936.
6. Blake, H. A., and Manion, W. C.: Thoracic arterial arch anomalies. *Circulation, 26*:251, 1962.
7. Blalock, Alfred: Surgical procedures employed and anatomic variations encountered in the treatment of congenital pulmonic stenosis. *Surg Gynecol Obstet, 87*:385, 1948.
8. Edwards, J.: Anomalies of the derivatives of the aortic arch system. *Med Clin North Am, 32*:925, 1948.
9. Ewald, W.: Einige falle von arcus aortae dexter. *Z Pathol, (Frankfurter), 34*:87, 1926.
10. Felson, B., and Palayew, M. J.: The two types of right aortic arch. *Radiology, 81*:745, 1963.
11. Gerber, N.: Congenital atresia of the subclavian artery. *Am J Dis Child, 113*:709, 1967.
12. Ghon, A.: Ueber eine seltene entwicklungstorung des gefassystems. *Verh Dtsch Ges Pathol, 12*:242, 1908.

13. Grollman, J. H.; Bedynek, J. L.; Henderson, H. S., and Hall, R. J.: Right aortic arch with an aberrant retroesophageal innominate artery: angiographic diagnosis. *Radiology, 90*:782, 1968.
14. Gruber, G. B.: Zwei falle von dextropositio des aortgenbogens. *Pathol (Frankfurter), 10*:375, 1912.
15. Hastreiter, A. R.: d'Cruz, I. A., and Cantez, T.: Right-sided aorta. *Br Heart J, 28*:722, 1966.
16. Keats, T. E., and Martt, J. M.: Tracheoesophageal constriction produced by an unusual combination of anomalies of the great vessels. *Am Heart J, 63*:265, 1962.
17. Klinkhamer, A. C.: *Esophagography in Anomalies of the Aortic Arch System.* The Netherlands, Williams & Wilkins, 1969, pp. 31-62.
18. Kommerell, B.: Verlagerung der osophagus durch seine abnorm verlanfende arteria subclavia dextra (arteria lusoria). *Fortschr Geb Roentgenstr Nuklearmed, 54*:590, 1936.
19. Levine, S.; Serfas, L. S., and Rusinko, A.: Right aortic arch with subclavian steal syndrome (atresia of left common carotid and left subclavian arteries). *Am J Surg, 111*:632, 1966.
20. Maranhao, V.; Gooch, A. S.; Ablaza, S. G. G.; Nakhjavan, F. K., and Goldberg, H.: Congenital subclavian steal syndrome associated with right aortic arch. *Br Heart J, 30*:875, 1968.
21. Mustard, W. T.; Trimble, A. W., and Trusler, G. A.: Mediastinal vascular anomalies causing tracheal and esophageal compression and obstruction in childhood. *Can Med Assoc J, 87*:1301, 1962.
22. Shuford, W. H.; Sybers, R. G., and Edwards, F. K.: The three types of right aortic arch. *Am J Roentgenol Radium Ther Nucl Med, 109*:67, 1970.
23. Shuford, W. H.; Sybers, R. G., and Schlant, R. C.: Right aortic arch with isolation of the left subclavian artery. *Am J Roentgenol Radium Ther Nucl Med, 109*:75, 1970.
24. Shuford, W. H.; Sybers, R. G., and Schlant, R. C.: Subclavian steal syndrome in right aortic arch with isolation of the left subclavian artery. *Am Heart J, 82*:98, 1971.
25. Stewart, J. R.; Kincaid, O. W., and Edwards, J. E.: *An Atlas of Vascular Rings and Related Malformations of the Aortic Arch System.* Springfield, Thomas, 1964, pp. 8-13, 124-219.
26. Stewart, J. R.; Kincaid, O. W., and Titus, J. L.: Right aortic arch: plain film diagnosis and significance. *Am J Roentgenol Radium Ther Nucl Med, 97*:377, 1966.
27. Victoria, B. E.; Van Mierop, L. H. S., and Elliott, L. P.: Right aortic arch associated with contralateral congenital subclavian steal syndrome. *Am J Roentgenol Radium Ther Nucl Med, 108*: 582, 1970.
28. Wychulis, A. R.; Kincaid, O. W., and Danielson, G. K.: Congenital vascular ring: surgical considerations and results of operation. *Mayo Clin Proc, 46*:182, 1971.

CHAPTER 6

DOUBLE AORTIC ARCH

Definition. This anomaly is characterized by the presence of two aortic arches. The ascending aorta arises anteriorly to the trachea and divides into two arches which pass to the right and to the left of the trachea and esophagus. The right common carotid and right subclavian arteries arise from the right arch. Similarly, the left common carotid and left subclavian arteries arise from the left arch.[2, 14] It is not possible for an innominate artery to be present in this anomaly.[14] The two arches join posteriorly to form the descending aorta. More often, the aorta descends on the left side rather than on the right and the right arch is usually the larger.[3, 11]

Classification. Double aortic arch may be classified into two types depending upon the patency of the two arches. In Type 1, both arches are patent and functioning. In Type 2, both arches are intact, but one arch is atretic.[13, 14]

DOUBLE AORTIC ARCH WITH BOTH ARCHES
FUNCTIONING
(TYPE 1)

Definition. In Type 1 double aortic arch, both aortic arches are patent and functioning.

Incidence and Clinical Significance. Double aortic arch with both arches functioning is by far the most common type of double aortic arch.[3, 5] This results in a constricting ring of vessels completely encircling the trachea and esophagus producing various degrees of obstruction. Of the arch anomalies resulting in a vascular ring, double aortic arch is the most important.[5, 9] There may be a history of respiratory difficulty dating from birth. Occasionally, patients with this malformation have no symptoms, and the anomaly is discovered incidentally on chest x-ray or at postmortem examination.

Double aortic arch rarely is accompanied by congenital anomalies of the heart.[3]

Development. In this anomaly, both arches in Edwards' hypothetical double aortic arch system persist, and all segments remain patent, resulting in a functioning double aortic arch.

Chest Roentgenography. In the young infant, the chest x-ray is usually normal as it may be difficult to detect the position of the aortic arch.[10] A right-sided descending aorta may be the only abnormality. In the lateral view, anterior displacement of the trachea at the level of the aortic arch is sometimes observed.

In the older patient, the chest x-ray shows a widened mediastinal shadow.[1] There may be a defect in the right side of the trachea suggesting a right aortic arch. The aorta usually descends on the left of the spine.

Bilateral and posterior compression defects are present on the barium-filled esophagus at the level of the aortic arches.[10] The defect on the right side of the esophagus is produced by the right arch. The narrowing on the left side of the esophagus results from extrinsic pressure from the left arch. The compression on the posterior esophagus is due to the retroesophageal aortic arch.

The frontal esophagogram, particularly with barium not too thick, may be informative as to which arch is retroesophageal. The retroesophageal right arch produces an oblique defect on the barium-filled esophagus running downward from right to left. When the left arch is retroesophageal, an oblique defect extending downward from left to right may be visible on the frontal esophagogram.

Angiographic Features. Contrast studies show the ascending aorta dividing into two separate arches, each giving rise to its respective brachiocephalic vessels. The aorta usually descends on the left side of the spine. In this instance, the right or posterior arch courses to the left behind the esophagus, is usually the higher of the two arches, and joins the anterior left arch to form the descending aorta. Occasionally, the descending aorta is on the right side of the spine. In this situation, the left arch swings posteriorly behind the esophagus to join the right arch, forming the descending aorta. In most patients, the right arch is the larger of the two arches.

Representative Cases

Case 1. Functioning double aortic arch.

This five-month-old infant was admitted with the history of difficulty swallowing and noisy respirations with stridor since birth. Routine chest roentgenogram was normal. Barium swallow revealed a large posterior and bilateral compression defect on the proximal esophagus (Fig. 6-1 A & B). Angiocardiographic studies (Fig. 6-2 A & B) showed a double aortic arch with both arches well formed and functioning. The right arch gave rise to the right common carotid and right subclavian arteries, and the left common carotid and

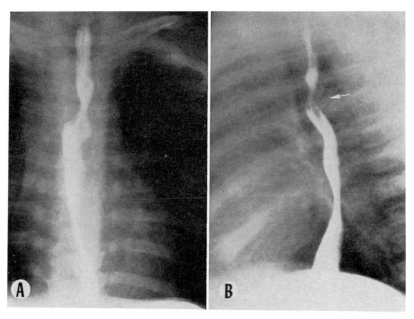

Figure 6-1. Case 1. Functioning double aortic arch. (A) Bilateral indentations on the barium-filled esophagus at the level of the aortic arches. (B) Lateral esophagogram reveals posterior compression of the esophagus (arrow). (From W. H. Shuford, R. G. Sybers, and H. S. Weens: The angiographic features of double aortic arch. *Am J Roentgenol Radium Ther Nucl Med, 116*:125, 1972.)

Representative Cases

left subclavian arteries originated from the left arch. The descending aorta was on the left side.

At surgery, a functioning double aortic arch was identified. Transection and ligation of the right arch just distal to the right subclavian artery was performed.

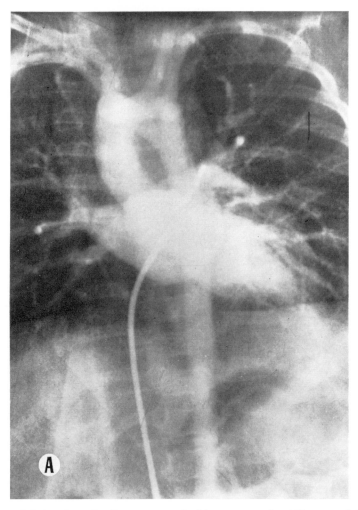

Figure 6-2 A. Case 1. Functioning double aortic arch. (A) Frontal levo-angiocardiogram shows the ascending aorta dividing into two arches with the descending aorta on the left side.

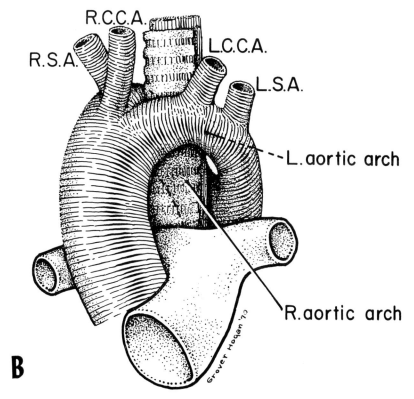

R.C.C.A.

R.S.A.

L.C.C.A.

L.S.A.

--L.aortic arch

R.aortic arch

B

Figure 6-2 B. Case 1. Functioning double aortic arch. (*B*) Diagram of angiogram. Each arch gives rise to its common carotid and subclavian arteries, respectively. (From W. H. Shuford, R. G. Sybers, and H. S. Weens: The angiographic features of double aortic arch. *Am J Roentgenol Radium Ther Nucl Med, 116*:125, 1972.)

Case 2. Functioning double aortic arch.

This seven-month-old male infant was admitted with a history of stridor and respiratory difficulty since birth. Chest roentgenograms disclosed clear lung fields and the heart and great vessels appeared to be normal. The esophagogram (Fig. 6-3) showed notch-like defects on both sides of the esophagus at the level of the aortic arch. There was an oblique indentation on the posterior portion of the esophagus coursing upward from left to right.

Angiocardiography (Fig. 6-4) demonstrated a normal ascending aorta which bifurcated into two arches of approximately equal size, each giving rise to its respective brachiocephalic vessels. The two arches joined posteriorly to form a left-sided upper descending aorta.

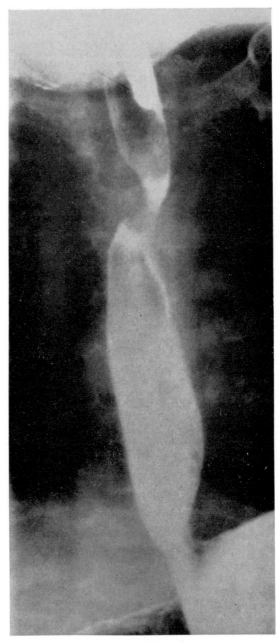

Figure 6-3. Case 2. Functioning double aortic arch. The esophagogram shows constriction of both sides of the esophagus at the level of the aortic arches.

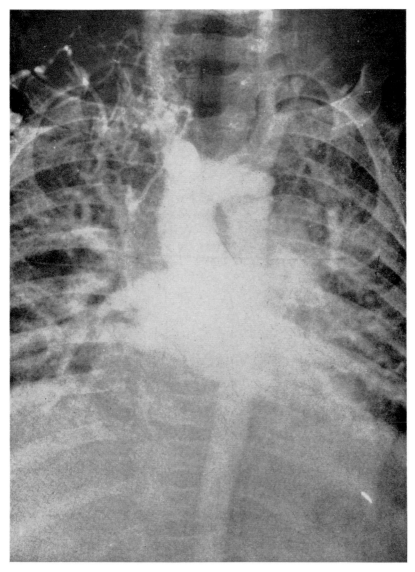

Figure 6-4. Case 2. Functioning double aortic arch. Frontal levoangio-cardiogram. The ascending aorta bifurcates into two arches of approximately equal size, each giving rise to a common carotid and a subclavian artery. The two arches join posteriorly to form a left-sided descending aorta.

Representative Cases

Case 3.   Functioning double aortic arch.

This thirty-seven-year-old woman gave a history of difficulty swallowing for years. Following thyroidectomy, she had laryngeal nerve paralysis and extensive scar formation. Her swallowing difficulties persisted and on admission plain chest films were normal. Barium esophagogram (Fig. 6-5 *A* & *B*) revealed a small pharyngeal pouch and some motor disturbances in swallowing. There was noted slight compression of the esophagus bilaterally and posteriorly at the level of the aortic arch and a vascular ring was suspected. Catheter aortography (Fig. 6-6) demonstrated a functioning double

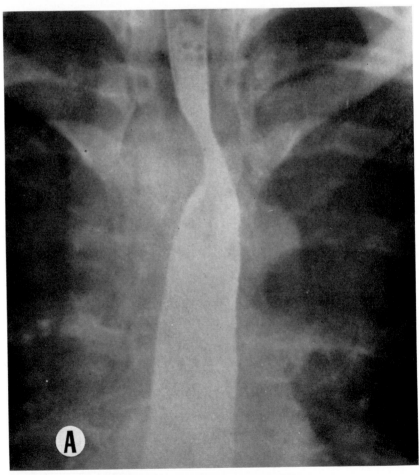

Figure 6-5 A.   Case 3.   Functioning double aortic arch.

aortic arch with the right brachiocephalic arteries arising from the right arch and the left brachiocephalic arteries originating from the left arch. The descending aorta was on the left side. Bronchoscopy was performed and showed no compression of the trachea. Because of the minimal esophageal compression demonstrated on the esophagogram, surgery was not performed.

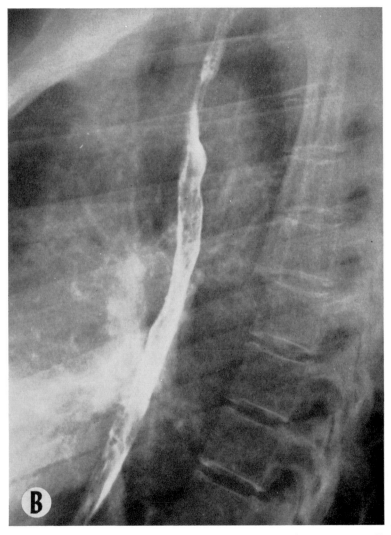

Figure 6-5 B. Case 3. Functioning double aortic arch. Barium swallow (*A* & *B*) reveals compression of the esophagus bilaterally and posteriorly at the level of the aortic arch suggesting the presence of a vascular ring.

Representative Cases

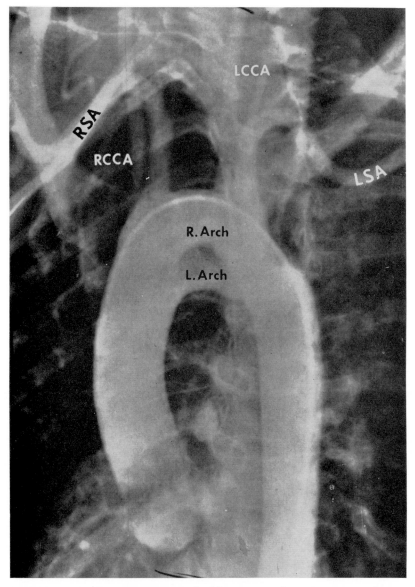

Figure 6-6. Case 3. Functioning double aortic arch. Left anterior oblique aortogram. The catheter passes from the descending aorta through the right arch to the ascending aorta. The right arch is larger and higher than the left arch. Each arch gives rise to its respective brachiocephalic vessels.

Case 4. Functioning double aortic arch.

Infant with symptomatic vascular ring. Chest roentgenograms (Fig. 6-7 *A* & *B*) revealed no abnormalities. Frontal and lateral esophagograms (Fig. 6-8 *A* & *B*) demonstrated bilateral and posterior compression defects of the barium-filled esophagus at the level of the aortic arches. Catheter aortography showed a right and left aortic arch, each giving rise to its respective brachiocephalic arteries. The descending aorta is left-sided (Fig. 6-9). (Courtesy of Dr. John A. Kirkpatrick.)

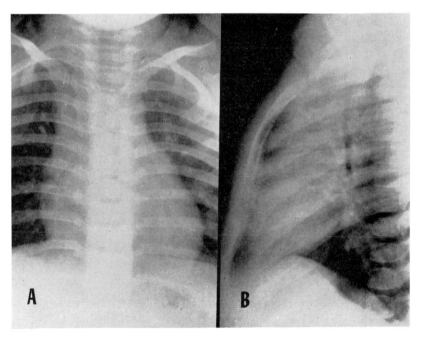

Figure 6-7. Case 4. Functioning double aortic arch. Frontal (*A*) and lateral (*B*) chest roentgenograms are normal. (Courtesy of Dr. John A. Kirkpatrick.)

Representative Cases

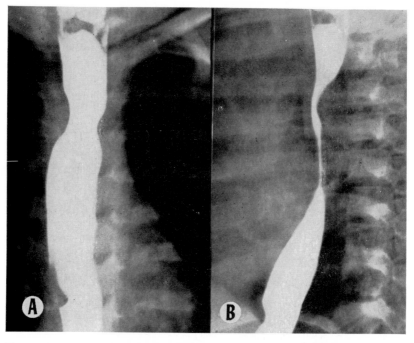

Figure 6-8. Case 4. Functioning double aortic arch. Frontal (*A*) and lateral (*B*) esophagograms demonstrate bilateral and posterior compression of the barium-filled esophagus at the level of the aortic arches. (Courtesy of Dr. John A. Kirkpatrick.)

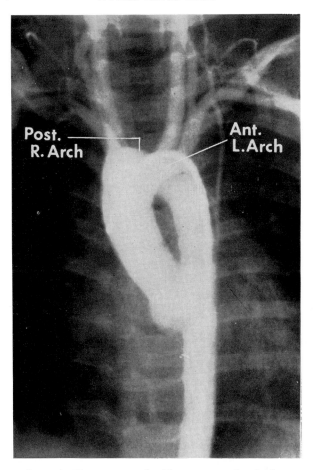

Figure 6-9. Case 4. Functioning double aortic arch. Catheter aortogram shows the ascending aorta dividing into a small anterior left arch and a large posterior right arch. Each arch gives rise to a common carotid and a subclavian artery. The aorta descends on the left side. (Courtesy of Dr. John A. Kirkpatrick.)

Representative Cases

Case 5. Functioning double aortic arch with hypoplastic left arch and right-sided descending aorta.

Infant with symptomatic vascular ring. Chest roentgenograms (Fig. 6-10 A & B) revealed only a right-sided descending aorta. The lateral barium-filled esophagogram demonstrated a prominent posterior compression defect (Fig. 6-11). Left ventriculography (Fig. 6-12 A & B) showed a normal ascending aorta dividing into two aortic arches, the left arch being considerably smaller than the right. Each arch gave rise to its respective brachiocephalic vessels. The aorta descended on the right side of the spine. (Courtesy of Dr. John A. Kirkpatrick.)

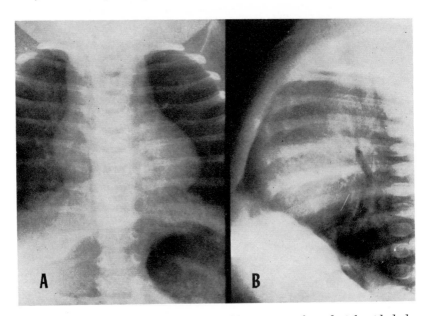

Figure 6-10. Case 5. Functioning double aortic arch and right-sided descending aorta. Frontal (A) and lateral (B) chest roentgenograms are normal except for the right-sided descending aorta. (Courtesy of Dr. John A. Kirkpatrick.)

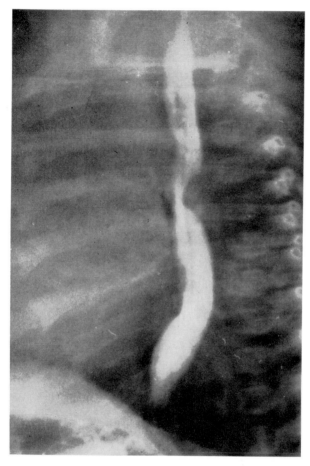

Figure 6-11. Case 5. Functioning double aortic arch and right-sided descending aorta. Lateral esophagogram reveals a localized posterior compression of the esophagus. (Courtesy of Dr. John A. Kirkpatrick.)

Representative Cases

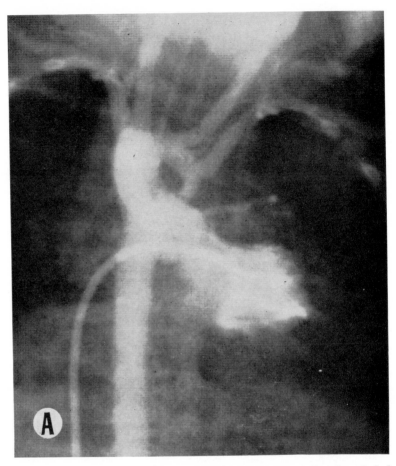

Figure 6-12. Case 5. Functioning double aortic arch and right-sided descending aorta. Frontal left ventriculogram (A) shows the ascending aorta dividing into a hypoplastic left arch and a large right arch. The two arches join posteriorly, and the descending aorta is right-sided. (Courtesy of Dr. John A. Kirkpatrick.)

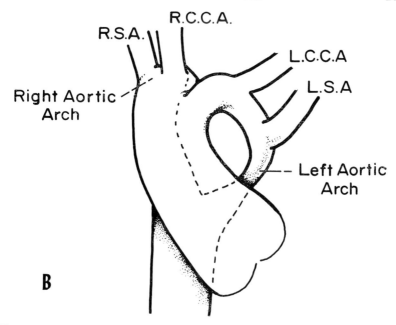

Figure 6-12. Case 5. Functioning double aortic arch and right-sided descending arch. (*B*) Diagram of angiogram. Each arch gives rise to its common carotid and subclavian arteries, respectively.

DOUBLE AORTIC ARCH WITH PARTIAL ATRESIA
OF ONE ARCH
(TYPE 2)

Definition. In this double aortic arch anomaly, both arches are in continuity. A segment of one arch is atretic and persists as a fibrous cord without a lumen.[13] The other arch is patent and functioning.

Hypothetically, atresia may involve either the right or left arch. However, there are no reported cases of atresia of the right arch.[14]

Theoretically, the atretic zone may be in one of four locations in the left arch, and we have classified double aortic arch with left arch atresia into four subtypes, depending upon the location of the atretic segment.[13] These sites of atresia are illustrated in Figure 6-13.

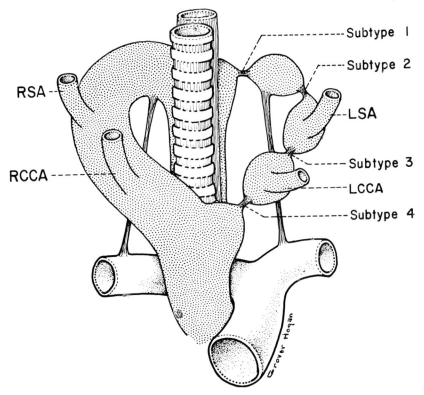

Figure 6-13. Classification of double aortic arch and atresia of the left arch. The four subtypes are illustrated. In Subtype 1, the atretic segment is between the left ductus arteriosus and the descendnig aorta. In Subtype 2, the atresia is between the left subclavian artery and the left ductus arteriosus. In Subtype 3, the atretic segment lies between the left common carotid and left subclavian arteries. In Subtype 4, the atretic zone is proximal to the origin of the left common carotid artery. (From W. H. Shuford, R. G. Sybers, and H. S. Weens: The angiographic features of double aortic arch. *Am J Roentgenol Radium Ther Nucl Med, 116*:125, 1972.)

Classification of Double Aortic Arch with Partial Atresia of Left Arch

Subtype 1. Atresia lies in the distal left arch between the left ductus arteriosus and descending aorta.

Subtype 2. Atresia is between the left subclavian artery and left ductus arteriosus.

Subtype 3. Atresia lies between the left common carotid and left subclavian arteries.

Subtype 4. Atresia involves the anterior portion of the left arch proximal to the origin of the left common carotid artery.

Subtype 1

Definition. In this double aortic arch malformation, the right arch is patent and functioning. The left arch is partially atretic, the atretic zone located between the descending aorta and the attachment of the left ductus arteriosus in the distal left arch.[4, 15, 16]

Incidence and Clinical Significance. This is a rare malformation of the aortic arch, and its true incidence is difficult to ascertain because of problems in diagnosis.[3] We have observed two proven cases with this arch anomaly. In both infants, symptoms of respiratory distress were present, necessitating double ligation of the atretic left arch.

Development. Double aortic arch, Subtype 1, results from partial regression of the left arch between the descending aorta and left ductus arteriosus. Both arches are in continuity, but this portion of the left arch becomes atretic and persists as a fibrous cord without a lumen (Fig. 6-14).

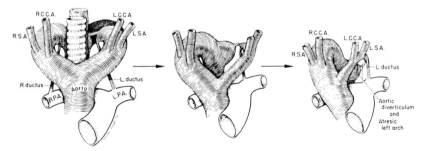

Figure 6-14. Development of double aortic arch with atresia of the left arch (Subtype 1). The atretic segment is distal to the left ductus arteriosus which connects to the left subclavian artery. A portion of the left arch between the left ductus arteriosus and descending aorta (shaded area) has undergone partial regression. (From W. H. Shuford, R. G. Sybers, and H. S. Weens: The angiographic features of double aortic arch. *Am J Roentgenol Radium Ther Nucl Med, 116*:125, 1972.)

Chest Roentgenography. The plain chest roentgenogram may disclose a right aortic arch and a right descending aorta. Barium studies of the esophagus show a compression defect on both the right and left sides of the esophagus with an indentation visible on the posterior esophageal wall.

Angiographic Features. Contrast studies reveal opacification of a right aortic arch and a right descending aorta. The first branch of the ascending aorta gives rise to the left common carotid and left subclavian arteries. The right common carotid and right subclavian arteries arise from the right aortic arch. A diverticulum-like structure may be present on the left lateral aspect of the distal right arch.

Differential Diagnosis. Right aortic arch with mirror-image branching (Figs. 5-2 and 5-9)[12] and double aortic arch with partial atresia of the left arch (Subtypes 1 and 2) (Fig. 6-13) will all show similar angiographic features.[13] The problem of differentiating these arch malformations is discussed in Chapter 7.

Representative Cases

Case 6. Double aortic arch with atresia of the left arch distal to the left ductus (Subtype 1). A nine-week-old male was found to have a heart murmur at birth. Cardiac catheterization showed the presence of a ventricular septal defect and mild pulmonary valvular stenosis. At seven weeks of age, he suddenly developed wheezing, cough, stridor, which was relieved by extending the head and neck. Plain chest roentgenogram was unremarkable. Barium studies showed constriction of the esophagus at the level of the aortic arch (Fig. 6-15 A & B). A levoangiocardiogram (Fig. 6-16 A, B, C) revealed the presence of a right-sided aortic arch and an aortic diverticulum of the descending aorta. The first branch of the right arch was interpreted to be the left innominate artery followed by the right common carotid and right subclavian arteries. From the roentgenographic findings the impression was right aortic arch with mirror-image branching and a left ligamentum arteriosum connecting to the diverticulum of the descending aorta thus forming a vascular ring.

Thoracotomy revealed the presence of a double aortic arch with the anterior arch the smaller of the two arches. The distal left arch was atretic beyond the left ligamentum arteriosum. The proximal portion of the left arch was patent and gave rise to the left common carotid and left subclavian arteries. The ligamentum arteriosum extended from the left pulmonary artery to the left subclavian artery. The distal left arch joined the descending aorta at the site of a diverticulum-like structure.

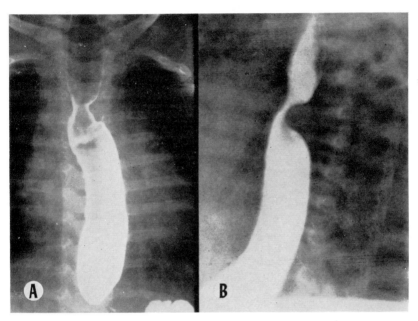

Figure 6-15. Case 6. Double arch with left arch atresia (Subtype 1). (A) There is narrowing of the esophagus from both the right and left sides due to pressure from the two arches. (B) A large retroesophageal defect is visible on the lateral esophagogram. (From W. H. Shuford, R. G. Sybers, and H. S. Weens: The angiographic features of double aortic arch. *Am J Roentgenol Radium Ther Nucl Med, 116*:125, 1972.)

Representative Cases

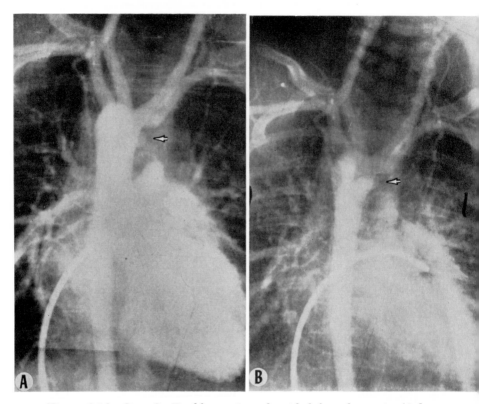

Figure 6-16. Case 6. Double aortic arch with left arch atresia (Subtype 1). (*A* & *B*) Levoangiocardiograms show right aortic arch and right-sided descending aorta. Left common carotid and left subclavian arteries appear to arise as a common trunk from the right arch. An aortic diverticulum projects from the left side of the distal right arch (arrow).

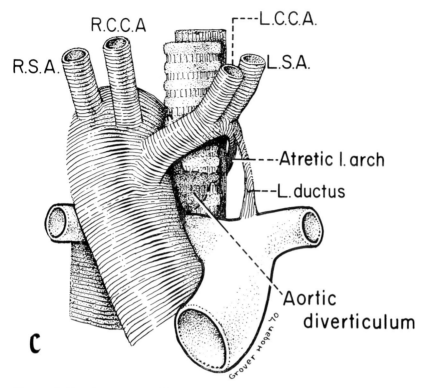

Figure 6-16. Case 6. Double aortic arch with left arch atresia (Subtype 1). (*C*) Drawing of vascular ring found at operation. The patent proximal portion of the left arch gives rise to the left common carotid and left sub-clavian arteries. The distal left arch is atretic and connects the left sub-clavian artery to an aortic diverticulum. The left ductus arteriosus extends between the left subclavian artery and the pulmonary artery. (From W. H. Shuford, R. C. Sybers, and H. S. Weens: The angiographic features of double aortic arch. *Am J Roentgenol Radium Ther Nucl Med, 116*:125, 1972.)

Case 7. Double aortic arch with atresia of left arch distal to left ductus (Subtype 1). An eight-day-old infant was admitted with persistent respiratory distress and stridor. Chest roentgenogram was within normal limits. Barium studies of the esophagus (Fig. 6-17) showed posterior indentation on the lateral view and in the frontal projection there was bilateral notching at the level of the aortic arch. A levoangiocardiogram (Fig. 6-18 A) revealed a right-sided aortic arch and a right descending aorta. The left common carotid and left subclavian arteries appeared to have a common origin from the aorta. The right common carotid and right subclavian arteries originated as separate branches from the right arch. A diverticulum-like structure was present on the left lateral aspect of the distal right arch and was particularly prominent on the right anterior oblique retrograde aortogram (Fig. 6-18 *B*). From the roentgenographic findings, the impression was right aortic arch with mirror-image branching and a left ligamentum arteriosum connecting to the diverticulum of the descending aorta thus forming a vascular ring.

Thoracotomy revealed a double aortic arch with the ascending aorta in normal position. The anterior arch was the smaller of the two arches. It crossed the midline giving rise to the left common carotid and left subclavian arteries. The left arch distal to the left ductus arteriosus was a cord-like structure and attached to the diverticulum of the descending aorta. The right common carotid and right subclavian arteries originated from the posterior right arch (Fig. 6-19 *A* & *B*).

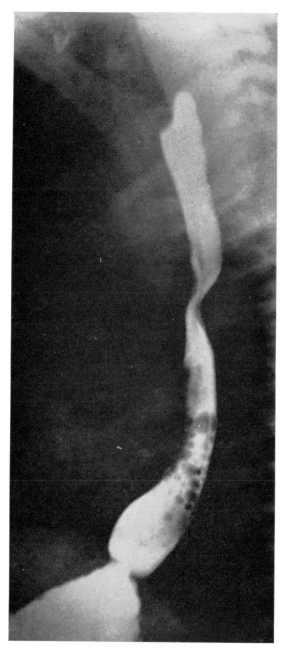

Figure 6-17. Case 7. Double aortic arch with left atresia (Subtype 1).
Barium studies of the esophagus show posterior indentation on the lateral
view.

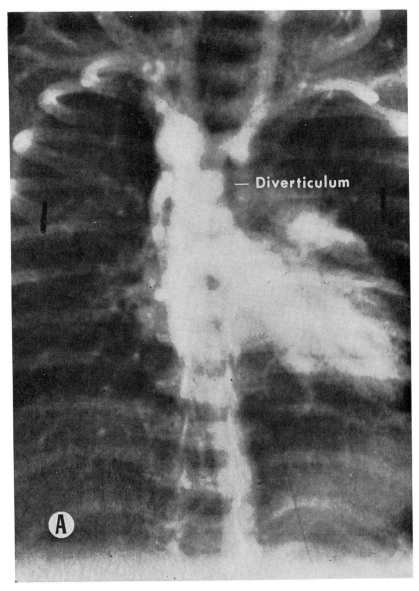

Figure 6-18. Case 7. Double aortic arch with left arch atresia (Subtype 1). (A) Levoangiocardiogram shows a right-sided aortic arch and a right descending aorta. The left common carotid and left subclavian arteries appear to have a common origin from the aorta. The right common carotid and right subclavian arteries arise as separate branches from the right arch.

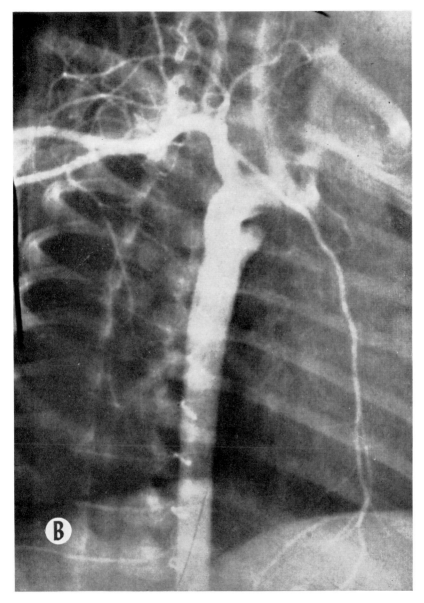

Figure 6-18. Case 7. Double aortic arch with left arch atresia (Subtype 1). (*B*) An aortic diverticulum is visible on the left lateral aspect of the distal right arch and is particularly prominent on the right anterior oblique retrograde aortogram.

Representative Cases

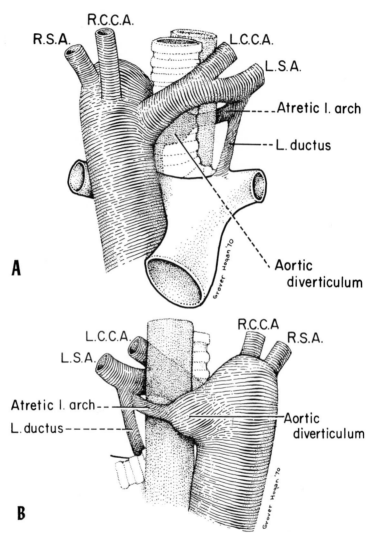

Figure 6-19. Case 7. Double aortic arch with left arch atresia (Subtype 1). Drawing of vascular ring. Frontal (*A*) and posterior (*B*) views show the smaller left arch giving rise to a left common carotid artery and left subclavian artery. The distal left arch is atretic beyond the left ductus arteriosus and connects to an aortic diverticulum.

Subtype 2

Definition. In this double aortic arch malformation, the right arch is patent and functioning. The left arch is partially atretic, the atretic zone located between the left ductus arteriosus and the left subclavian artery.[4]

Incidence and Clinical Significance. This is a rare type of double aortic arch anomaly, and its true incidence is difficult to ascertain because of problems in diagnosis. We have studied three cases with this malformation. In each instance, symptoms of respiratory distress necessitated surgical intervention.

Development. Double aortic arch Subtype 2 results from partial regression of the left arch between the left ductus arteriosus and the left subclavian artery. Both arches are in continuity but this portion of the left arch becomes atretic and persists as a fibrous cord without a lumen (Fig. 6-20).

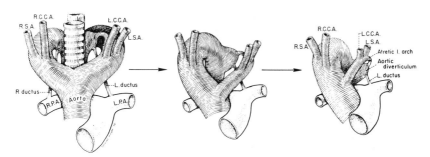

Figure 6-20. Development of double aortic arch with atresia of the left arch (Subtype 2). A portion of the left arch between the left subclavian artery and the left ductus arteriosus (shaded area) has undergone partial regression. The left ductus arteriosus extends from the aortic diverticulum to the left pulmonary artery. (From W. H. Shuford, R. G. Sybers, and H. S. Weens: The angiographic features of double aortic arch. *Am J Roentgenol Redium Ther Nucl Med, 116:*125, 1972.)

Chest Roentgenography. The plain chest roentgenograms may disclose a right aortic arch and a right descending aorta. Barium studies of the esophagus reveal a compression defect on both the right and left sides of the esophagus with an indentation on the posterior esophageal wall on the lateral projection.[13]

Angiographic Features. Angiography reveals opacification of a right aortic arch and a right descending aorta. The first branch of the ascending aorta gives rise to the left common carotid and left subclavian arteries. The right common carotid and right subclavian arteries arise from the right aortic arch. A diverticulum-like structure may be visualized on the left lateral aspect of the distal right arch.

Differential Diagnosis. Right aortic arch with mirror-image branching (Figs. 5-2 and 5-9) and double aortic arch with partial atresia of the left arch (Subtypes 1 and 2) (Fig. 6-13) will all show similar angiographic features. The problem of differentiating these arch malformations is discussed in Chapter 7.

Representative Cases

Case 8. Double aortic arch with atresia of the left arch proximal to left ductus (Subtype 2). This five-month-old female developed pneumonia and respiratory distress. Frontal chest roentgenogram (Fig. 6-21 A) revealed clear lung fields. The heart was of normal size. A right aortic arch was present with a right-sided descending aorta. The frontal esophagogram (Fig. 6-21 B) showed the right arch to compress the right lateral wall of the esophagus with a notch-like defect in the left wall. On the lateral view, a large retroesophageal impression was visible. Frontal levoangiocardiogram (Fig. 6-22 A & B) showed the ascending aorta coursing upward to the right of the trachea and descending on the right side. The right common carotid and right subclavian arteries arose from the right arch. There was an overlap of the left common carotid and left subclavian arteries, and their site of origin could not be determined. A large outpouching was visible along the left lateral aspect of the distal right arch. From the roentgenographic findings the impression was right aortic arch with mirror-image branching and a left ligamentum arteriosum connecting to the diverticulum of the descending aorta, thus forming a vascular ring.

Surgical exploration revealed the presence of a double aortic arch and a diverticulum on the distal portion of the right arch from which a ligamentum arteriosum extended around the left side of the trachea and esophagus and inserted into the pulmonary artery. The anterior segment of the double arch was the smaller of the two arches, giving rise to the left common carotid and left subclavian arteries. From the left subclavian artery, an obliterated vascular channel coursed to the left of the trachea and esophagus and connected the left subclavian artery to the aortic diverticulum at the point of attachment of the left ligamentum arteriosum. The right common carotid and right subclavian arteries originated as separate branches from the posterior large right arch.

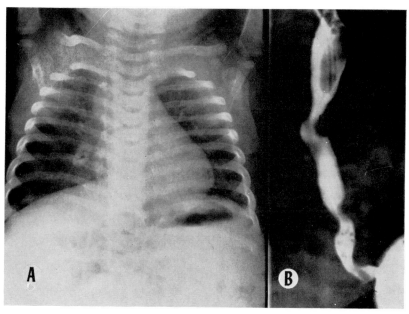

Figure 6-21. Case 8. Double aortic arch with left arch atresia (Subtype 2). (A) Chest roentgenogram shows a right aortic arch and a right descending aorta. (B) The frontal esophagogram reveals bilateral notch-like defects of the esophagus at the level of the aortic arch.

Representative Cases

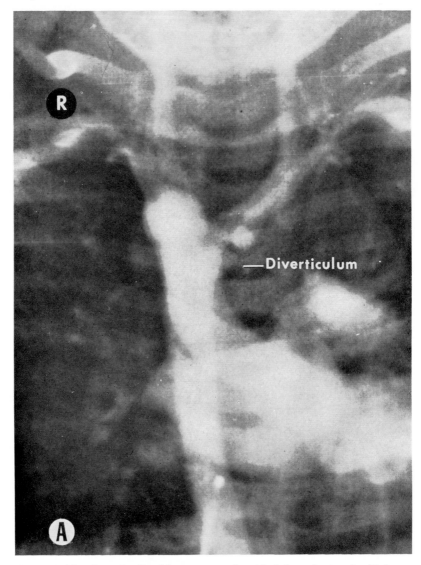

Figure 6-22. Case 8. Double aortic arch with left arch atresia (Subtype 2). (A) Levoangiocardiogram shows a large right aortic arch and right descending aorta with the right common carotid and right subclavian arteries arising from the right arch. The origins of the left common carotid and left subclavian arteries are not definite. An aortic diverticulum projects from the distal right arch.

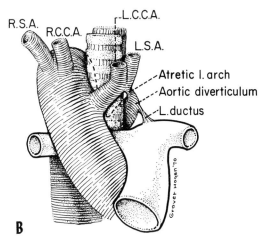

R.S.A. R.C.C.A. ┌-L.C.C.A.

L.S.A.

Atretic l. arch

Aortic diverticulum

L.ductus

B

Figure 6-22. Case 8. Double aortic arch with left arch atresia (Subtype 2). (*B*) Drawing of vascular ring found at operation.

Case 9. Double aortic arch with atresia of the left arch proximal to left ductus (Subtype 2). This three-month-old infant had respiratory stridor and difficulty with feeding since birth. Chest roentgenogram was negative except for the mediastinal configuration of a right aortic arch. Barium swallow revealed esophageal compression typical of a vascular ring. A levoangiocardiogram (Fig. 6-23 *A & B*) showed a large aorta which arched to the right of the trachea with a midline descending aorta. The right common carotid artery, right subclavian artery, left common carotid and left subclavian arteries all appeared to originate from the right arch. A prominent diverticulum-like structure protruded from the left upper descending aorta just above the level of the pulmonary artery. From the roentgenographic findings the impresssion was right aortic arch with mirror-image branching and a left ligamentum arteriosum connecting to the diverticulum of the descending aorta thus forming a vascular ring.

Thoracotomy revealed a vascular ring formed by a large right arch and a rudimentary anterior left arch. The left common carotid and left subclavian arteries arose from the patent proximal portion of the left arch. The distal portion of the left arch consisted of a stenosed vessel which connected the left subclavian artery to a diverticulum-like pouch on the descending aorta. The left ligamentum arteriosum ran from this aortic diverticulum to the pulmonary artery. The larger posterior right arch gave off the right common carotid and right subclavian arteries.

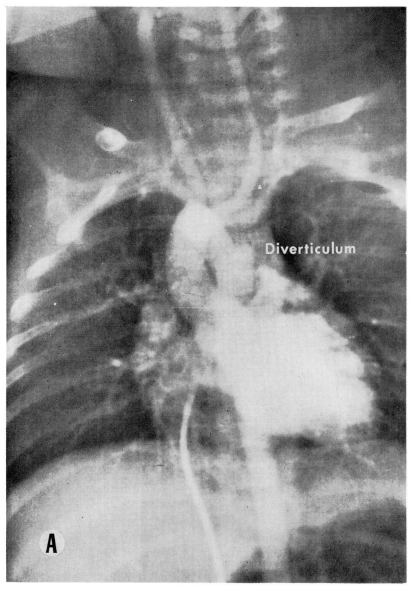

Figure 6-23. Case 9. Double aortic arch with left arch atresia (Subtype 2). (A) Levoangiocardiogram reveals a large aorta which arches to the right of the trachea with a midline descending aorta. The right common carotid, the right subclavian, the left common carotid and the left sub-clavian arteries all appear to originate from the right arch. A diverticulum-like structure protrudes from the left upper descending aorta.

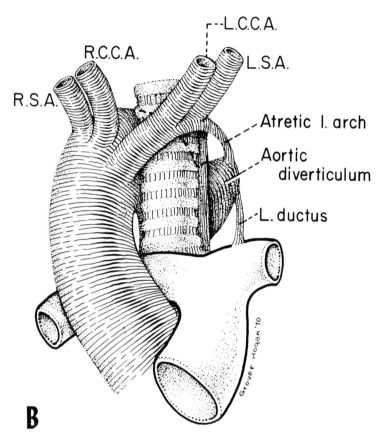

R.C.C.A.

L.C.C.A.

L.S.A.

R.S.A.

Atretic l. arch

Aortic
diverticulum

L. ductus

B

Figure 6-23. Case 9. Double aortic arch with left arch atresia (Subtype 2). (*B*) Drawing of vascular ring found at operation.

Subtype 3

Definition. In this double arch malformation, the right arch is patent and functioning. The left arch is partially atretic, the atretic zone located between the origins of the left subclavian artery and the left common carotid artery.

Incidence and Clinical Significance. This is an extremely rare malformation. Only a few cases have been reported.[7, 8] No examples of this malformation were observed in our series. A vascular ring is present, and symptoms resulting from tracheal and esophageal compression may be present.

Development. Double aortic arch Subtype 3 results from partial regression of the left arch between the left subclavian artery and the left common carotid artery. Both arches are in continuity, but this portion of the left arch becomes atretic and persists as a fibrous cord without a lumen (Fig. 6-24).

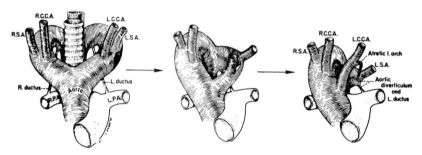

Figure 6-24. Development of double aortic arch with atresia of the left arch (Subtype 3). The atretic segment is between the origins of the left common carotid and left subclavian arteries. A portion of the left arch (shaded area) has undergone partial regression. (From W. H. Shuford, R. G. Sybers, and H. S. Weens: The angiographic features of double aortic arch. *Am J Roentgenol Radium Ther Nucl Med, 116*:125, 1972.)

Chest Roentgenography. The plain chest roentgenogram may disclose a right aortic arch. Barium studies of the esophagus show a compression defect on both the right and left sides of the esophagus with a filling defect in the posterior esophageal wall on the lateral view.

Angiographic Features. Angiography demonstrates opacification of a right aortic arch. The first branch of the ascending aorta is the left common carotid artery, followed by the right common carotid and right subclavian arteries. The fourth branch of the arch is the left subclavian artery arising from the upper descending aorta.

Differential Diagnosis. This condition cannot be distinguished roentgenographically from right aortic arch with an aberrant left subclavian artery (Chapter 7).

Subtype 4

Definition. In this double arch malformation, the right arch is patent and functioning. The left arch is partially atretic, the atretic zone located between the ascending aorta and the origin of the left common carotid artery.

Incidence and Clinical Significance. To our knowledge, there are no documented cases of this arch malformation. This malformation would result in a complete encirclement of the trachea and esophagus forming a vascular ring.

Development. Double aortic arch Subtype 4 would result from partial regression of the left arch between the ascending aorta and origin of the left common carotid artery. Both arches would be in continuity, but this portion of the left arch would become atretic and persist as a fibrous cord without a lumen (Fig. 6-25).

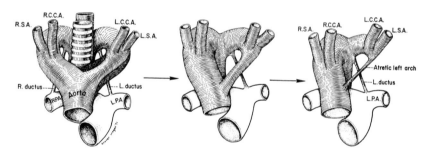

Figure 6-25. Development of double aortic arch with atresia of the left arch (Subtype 4). The atretic segment is between the left common carotid artery and the ascending aorta. A portion of the left arch (shaded area) has undergone partial regression.

Chest Roentgenography. The frontal chest roentgenogram should show a right aortic arch. Barium studies of the esophagus should show compression defects on both the right and left sides of the esophagus at the level of the aortic arch with a large posterior defect on the lateral esophagogram.

Angiographic Features. The right aortic arch should opacify with the first branch of the arch being the right common carotid artery, followed by the right subclavian artery. The third branch of the right arch should appear to be an aberrant left innominate artery giving rise to the left common carotid and left subclavian arteries.

Differential Diagnosis. This malformation could not be differentiated roentgenographically from right aortic arch with an aberrant retroesophageal left innominate artery (Chapter 7).

REFERENCES

1. Arkin, Aaron: Double aortic arch with total persistence of the right and isthmus stenosis of the left arch: a new clinical and x-ray picture. Report of six cases in adults. *Am Heart J, 11*:444, 1936.
2. Edwards, J. E.: Anomalies of the derivatives of the aortic arch system. *Med Clin North Am, 32*:925, 1948.
3. Ekstrom, G., and Sandblom, P.: Double aortic arch. *Acta Chir Scandinav, 102*:183, 1951.
4. Griswold, H. E., Jr., and Young, M. D.: Double aortic arch: report of two cases and review of the literature. *Pediatrics, 4*:751, 1949.
5. Gross, R. E.: Arterial malformations which cause compression of the trachea on esophagus. *Circulation, 11*:124, 1955.
6. Hallman, G. L.; Cooley, D. A., and Bloodwell, R. D.: Congenital vascular ring. *Surg Clin North Am, 46*:885, 1966.
7. Hurley, L. E., and Coates, A. E.: A case of right-sided aortic arch and persistent left superior vena cava. *J Anat, 61*:333, 1927.
8. Issajew, P. O.: Der doppelte aortenbogen. *Anat Anz, 73*:153, 1931.
9. Kirklin, J. W., and Clagett, O. T.: Vascular "rings" producing respiratory obstruction in infants. *Mayo Clin Proc, 25*:360, 1950.
10. Neuhauser, E.: The roentgen diagnosis of double aortic arch and other anomalies of the great vessels. *Am J Roentgenol Radium Ther Nucl Med, 56*:1, 1946.
11. Riker, W. L.: Anomalies of the aortic arch and their treatment. *Pediatr Clin North Am*, February 1954, pp. 181-195.
12. Shuford, W. H.; Sybers, R. G., and Edwards, F. K.: The three types of right aortic arch. *Am J Roentgenol Radium Ther Nucl Med, 109*:67, 1970.
13. Shuford, W. H.; Sybers, R. G., and Weens, H. S.: The angiographic features of double aortic arch. *Am J Roentgenol Radium Ther Nucl Med, 116*:125, 1972.
14. Stewart, J. R.; Kincaid, O. W., and Edwards, J. E.: *An Atlas of Vascular Rings and Related Malformations of the Aortic Arch System.* Springfield, Thomas, 1964, pp. 14-37.
15. Symbas, P. N.; Shuford, W. H.; Edwards, F. K., and Sehdeva, J. S.: Vascular ring: persistent right aortic arch, patent proximal left

arch, obliterated distal left arch and left ligamentum arteriosum. *J Thorac Cardiovasc Surg*, 61:149, 1971.

16. Wheeler, P. C., and Keats, T. E.: The left aortic diverticulum as a constricting vascular ring. *Am J Roentgenol Radium Ther Nucl Med*, 89:989, 1963.

CHAPTER 7

ROENTGENOLOGIC DIFFERENTIATION

BETWEEN DOUBLE AORTIC ARCH WITH LEFT

ARCH ATRESIA AND THE RIGHT AORTIC

ARCH MALFORMATIONS

THERE ARE TWO TYPES of double aortic arch.[3, 4] In one type, both arches are patent and functioning. In the other type, a portion of one arch is atretic, the atretic segment existing as a fibrous cord without a lumen.[4] Theoretically, atresia may involve either the right or left arch. In all reported cases, the atretic zone has been in the left arch.[4] Double aortic arch with left arch atresia may be divided into various subtypes depending upon the location of the atretic segment (Chaper 6).

The most precise method of studying double aortic arch malformations is angiography.[2] This method will readily identify the type when both arches are functioning. However, this method will not permit a definitive diagnosis of double aortic arch when the left arch is atretic.[3] This is true as it is impossible to distinguish between an atretic zone in one arch of a double aortic arch and complete interruption at this site by angiography.

Thus, for each subtype of double aortic arch with left arch atresia, there is a right aortic arch counterpart, and both have identical angiographic features. The study of the esophagus filled with barium offers valuable clues in differentiating some of the double aortic arch subtypes from the right aortic arch malformations.[1] However, there are some subtypes of left arch atresia which cannot be distinguished from their right aortic arch counterparts by roentgenologic means. This chapter will summarize the roentgenologic and angiographic features of double aortic arch with left arch atresia and the right aortic arch anomalies and emphasize points helpful in their differentiation.

Roentgenologic Differentiation between

A. Double aortic arch with left arch atresia (Subtype 1)
B. Type 1 right aortic arch (mirror-image branching—common type)

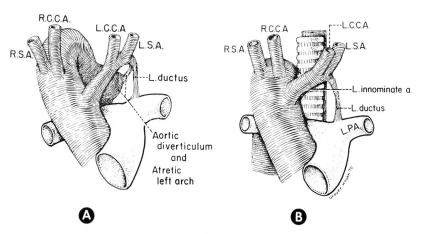

Figure 7-1. (A) Double aortic arch with left arch atresia (Subtype 1). (B) Type 1 right aortic arch (mirror-image branching—common type).

1. Angiography in both conditions shows a right aortic arch with mirror-image branching.
2. A vascular ring is present in double aortic arch (Subtype 1). There is no vascular ring present in Type 1 right aortic arch (mriror-image branching—common type).
3. The esophagogram is helpful in distinguishing these two arch malformations.

Roentgenologic Differentiation between

  A. Double aortic arch with left arch atresia (Subtype 2).
  B. Type 2 right aortic arch (mirror-image branching—rare type).

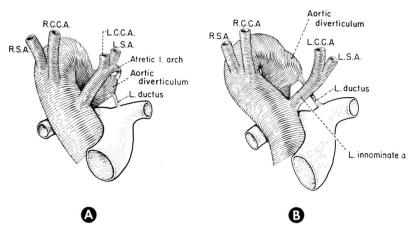

Ⓐ   **Ⓑ**

Figure 7-2. (A) Double aortic arch with left arch atresia (Subtype 2). (B) Type 2 right aortic arch (mirror-image branching—rare type).

In both conditions

1. Angiography shows a right aortic arch with mirror-image branching of the arch vessels. A posterior aortic diverticulum may be visualized.
2. A vascular ring is present.
3. Barium studies of the esophagus show a posterior compression defect in the lateral esophagogram.
4. These two anomalies cannot be distinguished from each other or from double aortic arch Subtype 1 by roentgenologic studies.

Thus, when angiography shows a right aortic arch with mirror-image branching in the presence of a symptomatic ring, the most likely diagnosis is double aortic arch with left arch atresia—because right aortic arch with mirror-image branching producing a vascular ring is extremely rare.

Roentgenologic Differentiation between

    A. Double aortic arch with left arch atresia (Subtype 3).

    B. Type 3 right aortic arch (aberrant left subclavian artery).

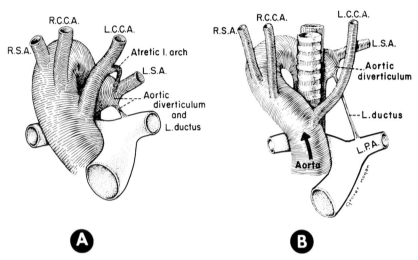

Figure 7-3. (A) Double aortic arch with left arch atresia (Subtype 3). (B) Type 3 right aortic arch (aberrant left subclavian artery).

In both conditions

1. Angiography shows a right aortic arch and an aberrant origin of the left subclavian artery.
2. A vascular ring is present.
3. Barium studies of the esophagus show a posterior compression defect on the lateral esophagogram.
4. These two anomalies cannot be distinguished from each other by roentgenologic studies.

When angiography shows a right aortic arch with an aberrant left subclavian artery, the most likely diagnosis is right aortic arch—because double aortic arch Subtype 3 is extremely rare.

Roentgenologic Differentiation between

    A. Double aortic arch and left arch atresia (Subtype 4).

    B. Type 4 right aortic arch (aberrant left innominate artery).

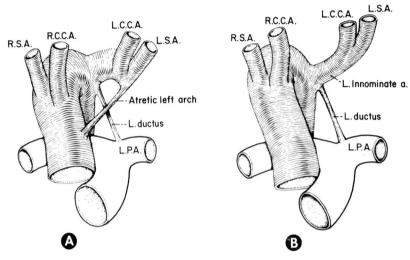

Figure 7-4. (A) Double aortic arch and left arch atresia (Subtype 4). (B) Type 4 right aortic arch (aberrant left innominate artery).

In both conditions

1. Angiography shows a right aortic arch with an aberrant left innominate artery.
2. A vascular ring is present.
3. Barium studies of the esophagus show a posterior constriction defect on the lateral esophagogram.
4. These two anomalies cannot be distinguished from each other by roentgenologic studies.

The right aortic arch anomaly is extremely rare, and the double aortic arch malformation remains a hypothetical possibility.

SUMMARY

1. When angiography shows a right aortic arch with mirror-image branching in the presence of a symptomatic vascular ring, the most likely diagnosis is double aortic arch with left arch atresia—because right aortic arch with mirror-image branching producing a vascular ring is extremely rare.
2. When angiography shows a right aortic arch with an aberrant left subclavian artery, the most likely diagnosis is right aortic

arch—because double aortic arch Subtype 3 is extremely rare.

3. When angiography shows a right aortic arch with an aberrant left innominate artery, it may be either Type 4 right aortic arch or Subtype 4 double aortic arch. However, both conditions are extremely rare. Only one case of the right aortic arch anomaly has been described, and to our knowledge there are no reported cases of the double aortic arch malformation.

REFERENCES

1. Ekstrom, G., and Sandblom, P.: Double aortic arch. *Acta Chir Scandinav, 102*:183, 1951.
2. Hallman, G. L.; Cooley, D. A., and Bloodwell, R. D.: Congenital vascular ring. *Surg Clin North Am, 46*:885, 1966.
3. Shuford, W. H.; Sybers, R. G., and Weens, H. S.: The angiographic features of double aortic arch. *Am J Roentgenol Radium Ther Nucl Med, 116*:125, 1972.
4. Stewart, J. R.; Kincaid, O. W., and Edwards, J. E.: *An Atlas of Vascular Rings and Related Malformations of the Aortic Arch System.* Springfield, Thomas, 1964, pp. 14-37.

CHAPTER 8

VASCULAR ANOMALIES OF THE MEDIASTINUM

CAUSING COMPRESSION OF THE TRACHEA

AND ESOPHAGUS

VASCULAR MALFORMATIONS in the superior madiastinum may compress the trachea and esophagus and cause respiratory distress and difficulty swallowing.[3, 4, 5]

Although these malformations are many, only a few assume clinical importance. In this chapter we will discuss those vascular anomalies most often encountered at surgery. These are (a) the double aortic arch, (b) right aortic arch and aberrant left subclavian artery, (c) anomalous left pulmonary artery and (d) anomalous innominate artery.[4, 7, 9]

THE ROENTGENOLOGICAL EXAMINATION

The radiologic examination of the mediastinum is the most important means of recognizing these conditions. Although chest roentgenograms are frequently normal, particularly in the young infant, one may see a right aortic arch and there may be indentation on the walls of the trachea. Barium studies of the esophagus provide the most important diagnostic clues. Roentgenographic demonstration of compression defects on the barium-filled esophagus may be diagnostic of a vascular ring (Figs. 6-1, 6-3, 6-8). If more conclusive information is desired, contrast studies of the heart and great vessels may delineate the precise vascular malformation. (Figs. 6-2 (A), 6-9 and 6-12 (A).

In our experience, angiocardiography, either by the intravenous method or selective injection into the heart or pulmonary artery, has been the most satisfactory method of studying patients with suspected vascular ring. This technique will identify the rare aberrant left pulmonary artery. Also, on the levoangiographic phase there is satisfactory opacification of the aorta and associated arch vessels. While catheter aortography may provide a higher degree of opacification of the aorta, in infants it is often difficult to introduce a catheter of sufficient size to deliver an adequate bolus of contrast media. In some cases when the angiographic findings are equivocal, we have employed countercurrent brachial arteriography to better visualize the origin of the subclavian arteries. However, as an initial examination this procedure is somewhat unsatisfactory, as it usually fails to completely outline the arterial malformation, particularly both limbs of the double aortic arch. Irrespective of which technique is employed, the anteroposterior study has been more reliable and has provided more information than the oblique or lateral projections.

DOUBLE AORTIC ARCH

By far the most common malformation of the aortic arch system requiring surgical treatment is the double aortic arch.[3, 4, 5, 9] In most series, double aortic arch with both arches patent is the most common type.[3, 5, 9] However, in our experience, double aortic arch with left arch atresia was slightly more common than double aortic arch with both arches functioning.

Contrast studies of the aorta readily identify the functioning double aortic arch (Fig. 6-2). When the left arch is atretic, angiography may be misleading, showing a right aortic arch and a diverticulum of the upper descending aorta (Figs. 6-16, 6-18, 6-22, 6-23). Initially, we erroneously believed these cases to be examples of what has been referred to as right aortic arch and a left-sided ligamentum arteriosum.[3, 4, 5] However, at surgery, all were proven to have a double aortic arch with the left arch atretic.

RIGHT AORTIC ARCH AND ABERRANT LEFT
SUBCLAVIAN ARTERY

Right aortic arch and an aberrant left subclavian artery is the most common malformation of the aortic arch system which completely encircles the trachea and esophagus.[7] A vascular ring is formed by the aortic arch on the right, posteriorly by the retro-esophageal aortic arch or the left subclavian artery, a ligamentum arteriosum on the left and the pulmonary artery anteriorly (Fig. 5-13, 5-14). Usually, however, this vascular ring is sufficiently loose that there is little or no encroachment upon the trachea or the esophagus.[7, 9] Of the patients requiring surgery at this hospital for a symptomatic vascular ring, none were found to have a right aortic arch and aberrant left subclavian artery. In our experience, when these patients are studied angiographically, it is because of an abnormal mediastinal configuration on the chest roentgenogram, or because of the associated cardiac malformation.

Contrast studies of the aorta reveal a right aortic arch and the aberrant origin of the left subclavian artery, either from the descending aorta directly, or from an aortic diverticulum, as the fourth branch of the distal arch (Figs. 5-16, 5-17, 5-18, 5-19).

Rarely, the proximal portion of the aberrant left subclavian artery may be atretic or tightly stenotic (Fig. 5-39). When there is atresia, or when stenosis is sufficiently severe, the left subclavian artery does not opacify from the aorta, but receives blood by collateral flow through the left vertebral artery. The angiographic findings (Fig. 5-42) are similar to those of right aortic arch with isolation of the left subclavian artery (Figs. 5-29, 5-32, 5-37). Patients with a right aortic arch and an atretic aberrant left subclavian artery may have a symptomatic vascular ring,[1, 6, 8] and can be differentiated from right aortic arch with isolation of the left subclavian artery by the retroesophageal defect on the lateral esophagogram.

ANOMALOUS LEFT PULMONARY ARTERY

This is a rare vascular anomaly. In this malformation, the aberrant left pulmonary artery arises to the right of the trachea, passing between the trachea and the esophagus. The trachea is thus compressed anteriorly by the main pulmonary artery, and posteriorly by the aberrant pulmonary vessel (Fig. 8-2).[2]

The clinical picture is similar to that produced by the more commonly encountered aortic arch anomalies.[2]

Barium studies of the esophagus are most helpful in the diagnosis of this vascular malformation. Characteristically, the aberrant left pulmonary artery indents the anterior wall of the barium-filled esophagus close to the level of the carina.[2] Pulmonary angiography should be performed when this condition is suspected (Fig. 8-1).

Representative Case

This premature female infant (birthweight 3 lbs. 3 ozs.) had no difficulty until three-and-one-half months of age when she developed intermittent stridor which later was associated with choking, apnea and cyanosis.

Chest roentgenograms revealed no abnormality. Barium studies of the esophagus demonstrated a pulsating indentation of the esophagus on its anterior and left lateral aspect at the level of the carina suggesting the presence of an aberrant left pulmonary artery.

Right ventriculography revealed the left pulmonary artery to arise aberrantly from the right main pulmonary artery (Fig. 8-1).

At surgery, the left pulmonary artery emerged to the right of the trachea and was dissected free from its posterior aspect (Fig. 8-2). (Courtesy of Dr. Dwight C. McGoon.)

Representative Cases

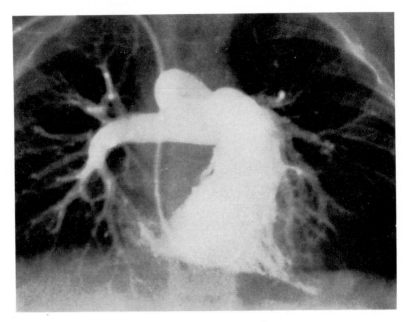

Figure 8-1. Case 1. Aberrant left pulmonary artery.

Right ventriculogram shows the left pulmonary artery to arise aberrantly from the right main pulmonary artery crossing to the left side between the trachea and esophagus and compressing the posterior wall of the trachea. (From P. M. Clarkson, D. G. Ritter, S. H. Rahimtoola, F. K. Hallermann, and D. C. McGoon: Aberrant left pulmonary artery. *Am J Dis Child, 113*:373, 1967.)

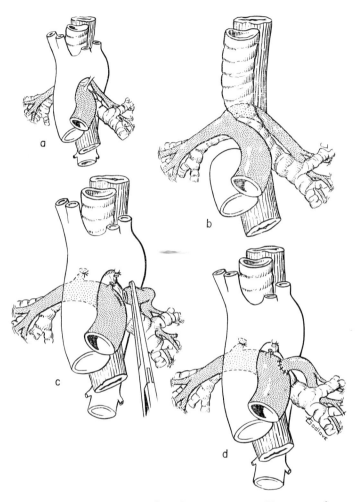

Figure 8-2. Case 1. Aberrant left pulmonary artery. Diagram of operative procedure. (a) Left pulmonary artery has aberrant origin. (b) Details of anomaly. Aorta removed. (c and d) Left pulmonary artery divided and brought from behind the trachea and anastomosed to the left side of the main pulmonary artery. (From P. M. Clarkson, D. G. Ritter, S. H. Rahimtoola, F. K. Hallerman, and D. C. McGoon: Aberrant left pulmonary artery. *Am J Dis Child, 113*:373, 1967.)

ANOMALOUS INNOMINATE ARTERY

In this anomaly, the innominate artery arises distally from the aortic arch and crosses in front of the trachea to the right side of the neck. The anomalous vessel may produce a tracheal compression causing respiratory distress.[4, 9] These infants are frequently misdiagnosed as having tracheomalacia. Esophageal atresia is often present.

The lateral chest roentgenogram may show anterior compression of the trachea.[4] Angiography will confirm the abnormal origin of the innominate artery.

REFERENCES

1. Antia, A. U., and Ottesen, O. E.: Collateral circulation in subclavian stenosis or atresia. *Am J Cardiol, 18*:599, 1966.
2. Clarkson, P. M.; Ritter, D. G.; Rahimtoola, S. H.; Hallermann, F. K., and McGoon, D. C.: Aberrant left pulmonary artery. *Am J Dis Child, 113*:373, 1967.
3. Ellis, H. F.; Clagett, O. T., and Kirklin, J. W.: Vascular rings produced by anomalies of the aortic-arch system. *Surg Clin North Am, 35:* 979, 1955.
4. Gross, R. E.: Arterial malformations which cause compression of the trachea or esophagus. *Circulation, 11*:124, 1955.
5. Hallman, G. L.; Cooley, D. A., and Bloodwell, R. D.: Congenital vascular ring. *Surg Clin North Am, 46*:885, 1966.
6. Keats, T. E., and Martt, J. M.: Tracheoesophageal constriction produced by an unusual combination of anomalies of the great vessels. *Am Heart J, 63*:265, 1962.
7. Stewart, J. R.; Kincaid, O. W., and Titus, J. L.: Right aortic arch: plain film diagnosis and significance. *Am J Roentgenol Radium Ther Nucl Med, 97*:377, 1966.
8. Victorica, B. J.; Van Mierop, L. H. S., and Elliott, L. P.: Right aortic arch associated with contralateral congenital subclavian steal syndrome. *Am J Roenegenol Radium Ther Nucl Med, 108*:582, 1970.
9. Wychulis, A. R.; Kincaid, O. W.; Weidman, W. H., and Danielson, G. K.: Congenital vascular ring: surgical considerations and results of operation. *Mayo Clinic Proc, 46*:182, 1971.

Chapter 9

CERVICAL AORTIC ARCH

Definition. In this anomaly, the ascending aorta arises normally from the left ventricle and extends in such a fashion that the aortic arch is situated high in the neck on either side.

Incidence and Clinical Significance. Twelve cases have been reported, two left-sided,[5, 11, 12] and ten cases with the aortic arch in the right side of the neck.[2, 3, 7-10, 13-15, 18]

In all cases, a pulsatile mass was present in the neck above the clavicle. The pulsating mass may be mistaken for an aneurysm of the subclavian, carotid or innominate artery.[2, 10] Symptoms of a vascular ring may be present or may develop.[2, 13, 15] There have been no reported examples of cervical aortic arch malformations associated with intracardiac congenital heart disease.

Anatomic Features. In the reported cases of cervical aortic arch, the branching of the arch vessels has been of several types. In the two cases of left cervical aortic arch, there was normal branching of the arch vessels in one patient.[11, 12] In the other, there were separate origins of the left external and internal carotid arteries, and an aberrant right subclavian artery.[5]

In most of the reported cases of right cervical aortic arch, the right carotid arteries arose as independent vessels.[2, 3, 8-10] In a few cases, the branching of the arch vessels is not well documented, but apparently in some of these the carotid arteries arose from a common trunk.[14, 15] In all cases of right cervical aortic arch, the left subclavian artery originated as the last branch of the aortic arch from the retroesophageal segment of the aorta.

Development. In the development of the cervical aortic arch, there are two anatomic features that require an explanation—namely, (a) the branching of the arch vessels and (b) the location of the arch in the neck.

Figure 9-1 shows Edwards' hypothetical double aortic arch consisting of an embryonic aortic arch on each side, with each arch giving rise to a common carotid and a subclavian artery.[6, 16, 17, 19] Interruption of either the right or left arch in this basic pattern can explain those cases of cervical aortic arch with the

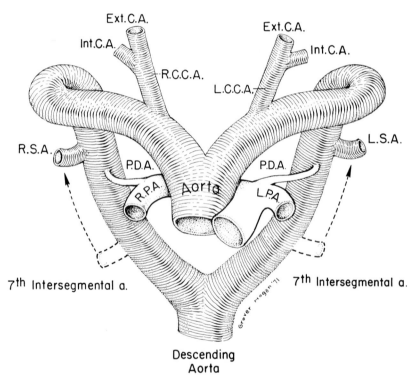

Figure 9-1. Hypothetical functioning double aortic arch with the carotid arteries arising from each arch as a common trunk. L.C.C.A. = left common carotid artery; R.C.C.A. = right common carotid artery; Int. C.A. = internal carotid artery; Ext. C.A. = external carotid artery; L.S.A. = left subclavian artery; R.S.A. = right subclavian artery; P.D.A. = patent ductus arteriosus; L.P.A. = left pulmonary artery; R.P.A. = right pulmonary artery. (From W. H. Shuford, R. G. Sybers, R. D. Milledge, and D. Brinsfield: The cervical aortic arch. *Am J Roentgenol Radium Ther Nucl Med, 116*:519, 1972.)

carotid arteries arising as a common trunk. Figure 9-2 shows the development of the case reported by Mahoney and Manning[12] and Lipchik and Young[11] (left cervical aortic arch with normal branching of the arch vessels).

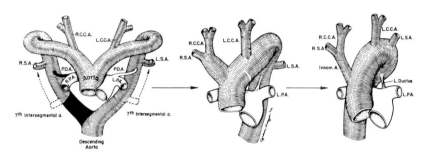

Figure 9-2. Development of left cervical aortic arch with normal branching of the arch vessels. There is interruption of the right embryonic arch between the right subclavian artery and descending aorta in the hypothetical double aortic arch with the carotid arteries arising as a common trunk. Areas in black indicate segments of complete regression. (From W. H. Shuford, R. G. Sybers, R. D. Milledge, and D. Brinsfield: The cervical aortic arch. *Am J Roentgenol Radium Ther Nucl Med, 116*:519, 1972.)

For an explanation of the development of the cases of cervical aortic arch with the carotid arteries arising as separate vessels, it is necessary to postulate a second type of hypothetical double aortic arch system, that is, a double aortic arch with the external and internal carotid arteries arising as independent vessels (Fig. 9-3). Figure 9-4 shows the result of interruption of the left embryonic arch between the left subclavian artery and the carotid arteries in this hypothetical pattern. A right aortic arch is formed, the first branch is the left common carotid artery, followed by separate origins of the right external and internal carotid arteries. The next branch is the right subclavian artery, followed by an aberrant left subclavian artery. Such is the branching of the arch vessels in most of the reported cases of right cervical arch.

Likewise, interruption of the right embryonic arch between the right subclavian artery and the carotid arteries in this hypothetical pattern (Fig. 9-5) explains the development of the one case of left cervical arch with independent origin of the carotid arteries.[5]

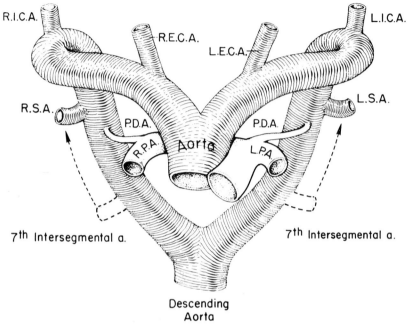

Figure 9-3. Hypothetical functioning double aortic arch with the external and internal carotid arteries arising separately from each arch. R.E.C.A. = right external carotid artery; R.I.C.A. = right internal carotid artery; L.E.C.A. = left external carotid artery; L.I.C.A. = left internal carotid artery. (From W. H. Shuford, R. G. Sybers, R. D. Milledge, and D. Brinsfield: The cervcial aortic arch. *Am J Roentgenol Radium Ther Nucl Med,* *116*:519, 1972.)

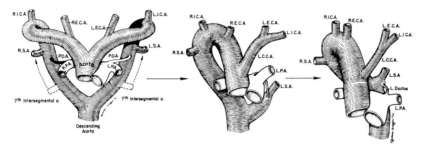

Figure 9-4. Development of right cervical aortic arch with the right internal and external carotid arteries arising as separate branches. There is interruption of the left embryonic arch between the left subclavian artery and the carotid arteries in the hypothetical double aortic arch with independent origin of the carotid arteries. The left common carotid artery is the first branch, followed by the right external carotid artery, the right internal carotid artery, the right subclavian artery and the left subclavian artery, in that order. Areas in black indicate segments of complete regression. (From W. H. Shuford, R. G. Sybers, R. D. Milledge, and D. Brinsfield: The cervical aortic arch. *Am J Roentgenol Radium Ther Nucl Med,* *116*:519, 1972.)

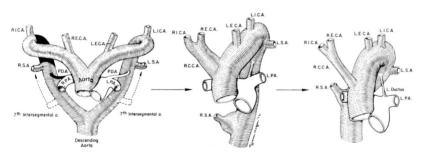

Figure 9-5. Development of left cervical aortic arch with the left internal and external carotid arteries arising as separate branches. There is interruption of the right embryonic arch between the right subclavian artery and the carotid arteries in the hypothetical double aortic arch with separate origin of the carotid arteries. Areas in black indicate segments of complete regression. (From W. H. Shuford, R. G. Sybers, R. D. Milledge, and D. Brinsfield: The cervical aortic arch. *Am J Roentgenol Radium Ther Nucl Med, 116*:519, 1972.)

The question as to which branchial arch forms the cervical aortic arch is of special interest. Normally, the fourth branchial arch forms the aortic arch [1, 4] (Chapter 1). However, the aortic arch may be derived from the second or third branchial arch,[2, 8, 12, 15] and we have shown in Figure 9-6 and Figure 9-7 the alterations in the Rathke diagram for the development of the aortic arch from the second and third branchial arches as well as from the fourth branchial arch.

There is a difference of opinion regarding the formation of the cervical arch. Those who believe that the cervical aorta is derived from the second[11, 12] or third[2, 8, 10] branchial arch point out that the location of the arch in the neck is evidence against its normal development and suggests persistence of a more cephalic branchial arch. Edwards, however, believes that the cervical aorta is formed normally from the fourth arch, but for some reason is retained abnormally in the neck.[13]

The independent origin of the carotid arteries in some cases of cervical aortic arch is also cited as further evidence that the cervical aorta is derived from the second or third branchial arch. This argument, however, is not necessarily valid. As shown in Figure 9-7, the aortic arch with independent origin of the carotid arteries may be derived from the fourth branchial arch as well as from the second and third branchial arches. At present, there appears to be no way of telling which of these possibilities is the correct one.

Chest Roentgenography. Nonspecific widening of the mediastinum may be the only abnormality. The trachea is usually displaced forward by the retroesophageal position of the distal arch. We have observed an oblique cutoff of the tracheal air shadow at the level of the thoracic inlet on the frontal projection due to the superimposition of the ascending aorta on its upward course to the neck. The aortic knob shadow is absent.

Barium studies of the esophagus show a posterior compression defect from the retroesophageal position of the distal arch. The esophagus may be displaced laterally in the neck by the cervical aorta.

Angiographic Features. The aortographic findings are striking. The aorta ascends into the neck, either to the right or left side, the apex of the arch makes a hairpin loop, and returns to the thorax, crossing the midline behind the esophagus, to descend along the spine opposite the side of the arch.

When the arch is right-sided, the left common carotid artery is the first branch and originates from the ascending aorta. The right external and internal carotid arteries usually originate as independent branches, although they may arise from a common trunk. The right subclavian artery is the next branch off the arch. The origin of the left subclavian artery is just distal to the retroesophageal segment of the aorta and may be from a conical diverticulum. In one case, the left subclavian artery was either isolated from the descending aorta, or was connected to the descending aorta by an atretic segment.[13]

In two reported cases of left-sided cervical aortic arch, the branching of the arch vessels was different. In the case of de Jong and Klinkhamer,[5] the right common carotid artery was the first branch of the ascending aorta followed by separate origins of the left external and internal carotid arteries. The left subclavian artery arose from the apex of the left arch, and the right subclavian artery had an aberrant origin as the last branch of the distal aortic arch.

The origin of the arch vessels in the case reported by Mahoney and Manning[12] (same case reported by Lipchik and Young[11]) apparently was identical to the branching of the normal left arch. The innominate artery was the first branch, followed by the left common carotid and left subclavian arteries.

Diagnosis. There have been no cases in which a correct diagnosis has been made prior to angiography. If one is aware of this rare arch anomaly, there are characteristic features which should permit its recognition.[3, 13]

Clinically, this anomaly should be suspected when one encounters a child with a pulsatile mass in the neck, with or without symptoms of a vascular ring. Compression of the neck mass may cause a decrease in heart rate, with diminution of the blood pressure in the opposite arm and legs.[13]

Barium studies of the esophagus may be most helpful, and previous reports have not emphasized the value of this examina-

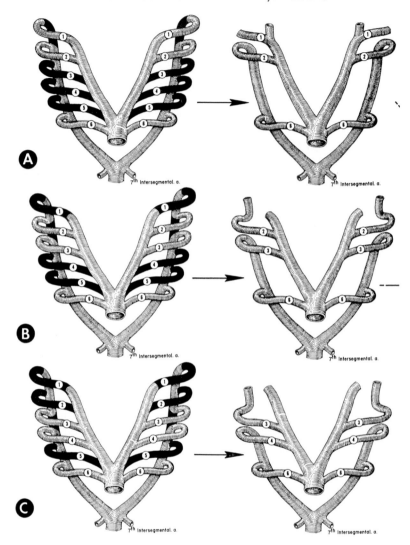

Figure 9-6. Alterations in the Rathke diagram for the development of a hypothetical double aortic arch with the carotid arteries arising from each arch as a common trunk. The theoretical development of the aortic arch in this hypothetical pattern from (A) the second branchial arch, (B) the third branchial arch and (C) the fourth branchial arch is shown. The six paired branchial arches are numbered. Areas in black indicate segments of regression. L.C.C.A. = left common carotid artery; R.C.C.A. = right common carotid artery; Ext. C.A. = external carotid artery; Int. C.A. = in-

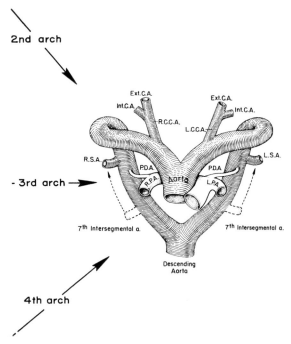

ternal carotid artery; R.S.A. = right subclavian artery; L.S.A. = left sub-
clavian artery. (From W. H. Shuford, R. G. Sybers, R. D. Milledge, and
D. Brinsfield: The cervical aortic arch. *Am J Roentgenol Radium Ther
Nucl Med, 116*:519, 1972.)

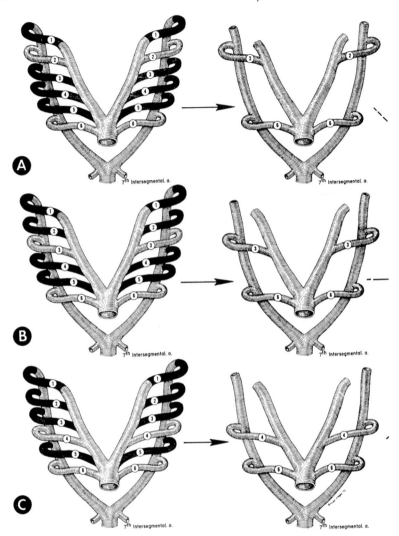

Figure 9-7. Alterations in the Rathke diagram for the development of a hypothetical double aortic arch with the internal and external carotid arteries arising separately from each arch. The theoretical development of the aortic arch in this hypothetical pattern from (A) the second branchial arch, (B) the third branchial arch and (C) the fourth branchial arch is shown. The six paired branchial arches are numbered. Areas in black indicate segments of regression. L.E.C.A. = left external carotid artery;

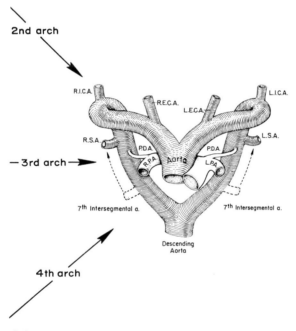

L.I.C.A. = left internal carotid artery; R.E.C.A. = right external carotid artery; R.I.C.A. = right internal carotid artery. (From W. H. Shuford, R. G. Sybers, R. D. Milledge, and D. Brinsfield: The cervical aortic arch. *Am J Roentgenol Radium Ther Nucl Med, 116:*519, 1972.)

tion in the diagnosis of cervical aortic arch. The large pulsating oblique defect just below the clavicles on the frontal view, with a prominent rounded indentation on the posterior esophageal wall on the lateral projection, identifies the retroesophageal course of the descending aorta. These findings, together with a pulsatile swelling in the neck, should be considered diagnostic of this arch anomaly. However, contrast studies of the aorta are necessary for a definite diagnosis.

Representative Cases

Case 1. Right cervical aortic arch. This seven-year-old girl was admitted to Grady Memorial Hospital for evaluation of a pulsatile mass in the right neck which was present since birth. Otherwise, the child was asymptomatic.

Physical examination revealed a thin girl in no distress. The pulse rate was 88 beats per minute. The blood pressure was 90/70 mm Hg reclining, 88/65 mm Hg in the sitting position. There was an approximately 2½ x 3 cm pulsatile swelling in the right neck just above the sternoclavicular joint. A harsh bruit was audible over the mass. The examination of the heart was negative.

Electrocardiogram was within normal limits. Chest roentgenogram (Fig. 9-8 A) showed the heart to be of normal size. The aortic knob shadow was absent. An oblique cutoff of the tracheal air shadow at the level of the thoracic inlet was visible. Lateral view of the chest (Fig. 9-8 B) showed the trachea to be displaced forward at the level of the aortic arch..

Barium studies of the esophagus (Fig. 9-9 A & B) revealed an obliquely directed defect running downward from right to left just below the level of the clavicles. On the lateral view, there was forward displacement of the esophagus at the same level. Aortography (Fig. 9-10 A, B, C) showed the arch of the aorta to lie in the right neck. The arch descended on the right to the level of T-4 at which point it crossed to the left of the spine. Below the level of T-6, the aorta descended in a normal fashion on the left side. The first branch of the ascending aorta was the left common carotid artery. The right external and internal carotid arteries arose separately from the apex of the arch. The right subclavian artery was the next vessel to arise from the arch. The left subclavian artery originated from a small conical diverticulum just distal to the retroesophageal segment of the aorta. Figure 9-11 shows the anatomy of the cervical aorta, its relation to the trachea and esophagus, and the branching of the arch vessels.

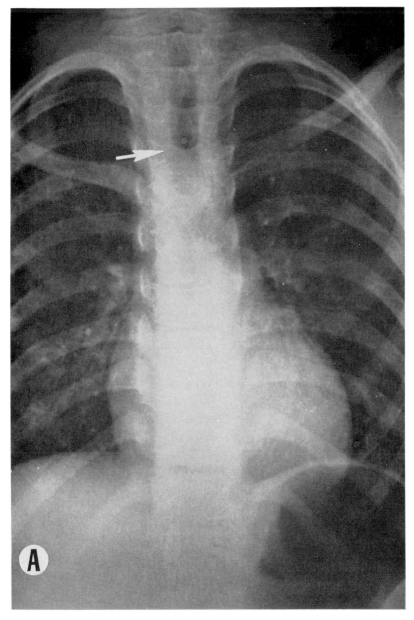

Figure 9-8. Case 1. Right cervical aortic arch. (A) The aortic shadow is absent. There is no widening of the mediastinum. The heart is normal in size. An oblique cutoff of the tracheal air shadow above the level of the clavicles is present (arrow).

Representative Cases

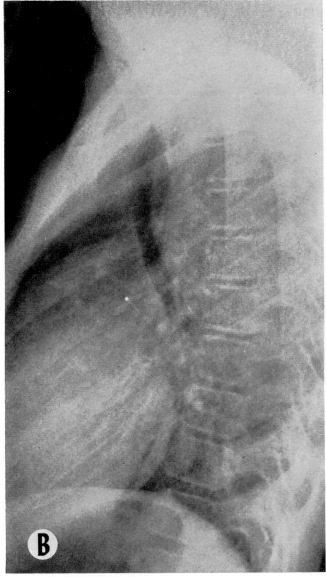

Figure 9-8. Case 1. Right cervical aortic arch. (*B*) On the lateral view, the trachea is displaced forward by the anomalously-placed aorta. (From W. H. Shuford, R. G. Sybers, R. D. Milledge, and D. Brinsfield: The cervical aortic arch. *Am J Roentgenol Radium Ther Nucl Med, 116:519,* 1972.)

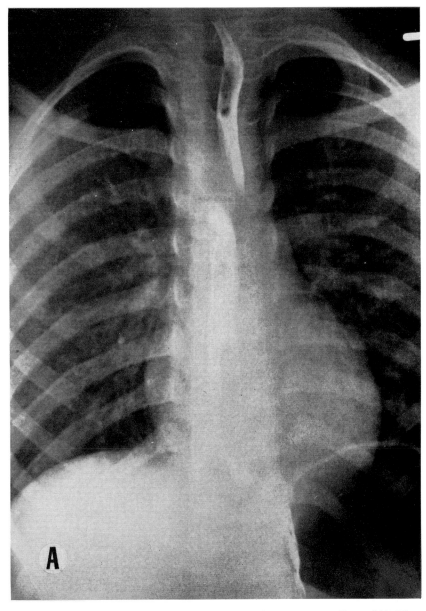

Figure 9-9. Case 1. Right cervical aortic arch. Barium swallow. (A) The retroesophageal aorta produces an oblique posterior compression defect on the esophagus.

Representative Cases

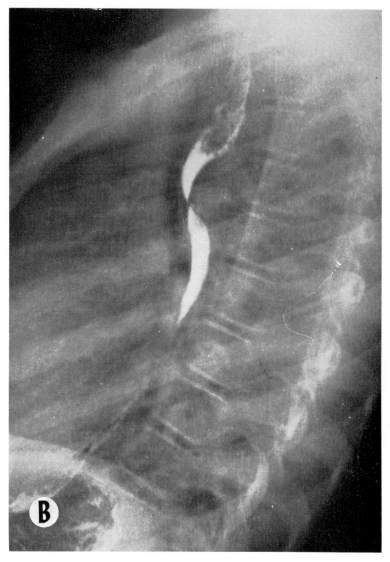

Figure 9-9. Case 1. Right cervical aortic arch. (*B*) The esophagus is displaced anteriorly by the aorta. (From W. H. Shuford, R. G. Sybers, R. D. Milledge, and D. Brinsfield: The cervical aortic arch. *Am J Roentgenol Radium Ther Nucl Med, 116*:519, 1972.)

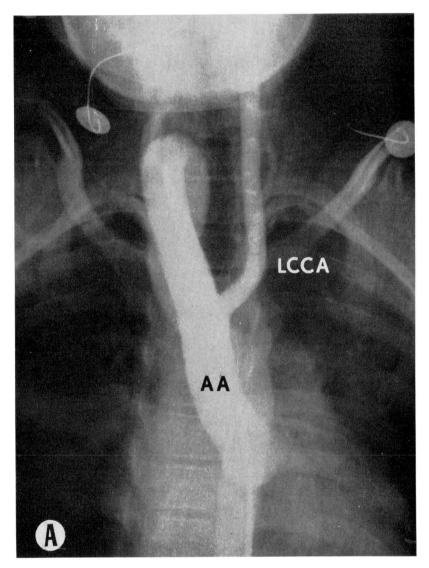

Figure 9-10. Case 1. Right cervical aortic arch. Thoracic aortogram. (A) The ascending aorta (AA) extends into the neck, to the right of the trachea. The first branch of the ascending aorta is the left common carotid artery. A.A. = ascending aorta; L.C.C.A. = left common carotid artery.

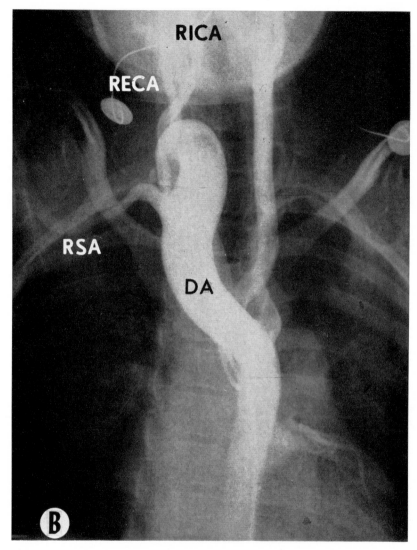

Figure 9-10. Case 1. Right cervical aortic arch. (*B*) One second later, the descending aorta (DA) is opacified. The right external and internal carotid arteries arise as separate branches from the apex of the arch. The right subclavian artery originates from the proximal descending aorta as the fourth branch. D.A. = descending aorta; R.I.C.A. = right internal carotid artery; R.E.C.A. = right external carotid artery; R.S.A. = right subclavian artery.

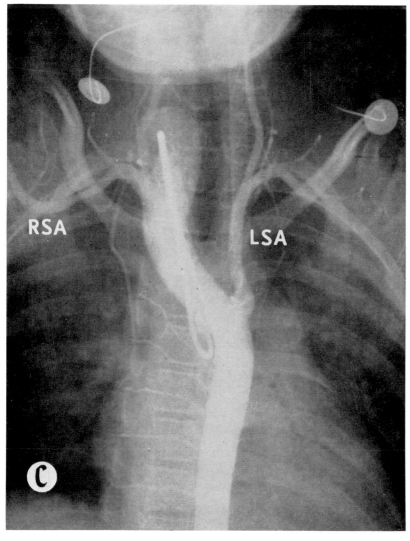

Figure 9-10. Case 1. Right cervical aortic arch. (*C*) The descending aorta crosses the midline behind the esophagus, to descend along the left side of the spine. The origin of the left subclavian artery is from a small conical diverticulum just distal to the retroesophageal segment of the descending aorta. L.S.A. = left subclavian artery. (From W. H. Shuford, R. G. Sybers, R. D. Milledge, and D. Brinsfield: The cervical aortic arch. *Am J Roentgenol Radium Ther Nucl Med, 116*:519, 1972.)

Representative Cases

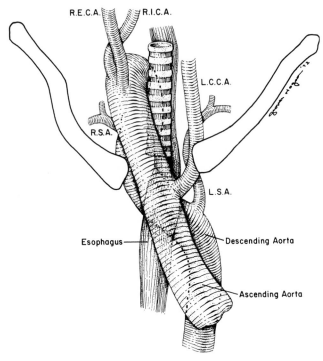

Figure 9-11. Case 1. Right cervical arch. The anatomy of the cervical aorta, its relation to the trachea and esophagus, and the branching of the arch vessels are shown. L.C.C.A. = left common carotid artery; R.E.C.A. = right external carotid artery; R.I.C.A. = right internal carotid artery; R.S.A. = right subclavian artery; L.S.A. = left subclavian artery. (From W. H. Shuford, R. G. Sybers, R. D. Milledge, and D. Brinsfield: The cervical aortic arch. *Am J Roentgenol Radium Ther Nucl Med, 116*:519, 1972.)

Case 2. Right-sided cervical aortic arch. This 2½-year-old child was hospitalized because of symptoms of tracheal and esophageal compression associated with a pulsatile mass in the right side of the neck.

On the chest roentgenogram, a vaguely outlined widening of the mediastinum to the right was present. Esophagograms (Fig. 9-12 *A* & *B*) revealed a large posterior compression defect typical of a retroesophageal vessel. The levoangiocardiograms (Fig. 9-13 *A* & *B*) showed a right cervical aortic arch. The oblique defect on the posterior aspect of the esophagus resulted from compression of the terminal portion of the aortic arch as it crossed from the right to the left side of the mediastinum. The branching of the arch vessels is as shown in Figure 9-14 *A* and *B*.

Surgical exploration was performed to relieve the tracheal and esophageal compression. Division of the left ligamentum arteriosum failed to alter significantly the number of pulmonary infections in this patient. (Courtesy of Dr. Melvin M. Figley.)

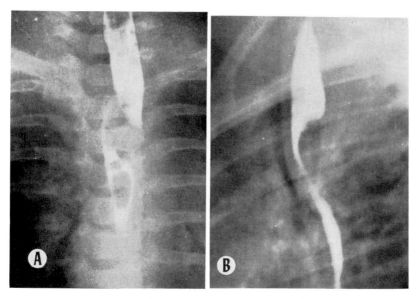

Figure 9-12. Case 2. Right cervical aortic arch. Esophagograms (*A* & *B*) demonstrate the retroesophageal aortic impression. (From L. W. M. Chang, E. L. Kaplan, D. Baum, and M. M. Figley: Aortic arch in the neck: a case report. *J Pediatr,* 79:788, 1971.)

Representative Cases

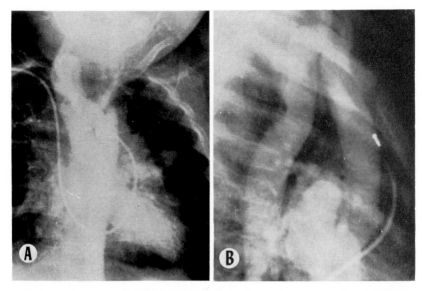

Figure 9-13. Case 2. Right cervical aortic arch. Levoangiocardiograms (*A* & *B*) show cervical position of right aortic arch. The first branch of the ascending aorta is the left common carotid artery, followed by the right external and internal carotid arteries. The fourth branch is the right subclavian artery with the left subclavian artery arising as the last branch of the arch. (From L. W. M. Chang, E. L. Kaplan, D. Baum, and M. M. Figley: Aortic arch in the neck: a case report. *J Pediatr,* 79:788, 1971.)

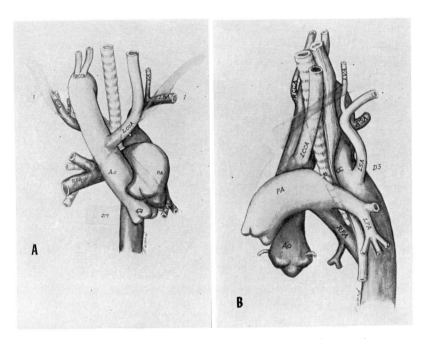

Figure 9-14. (*A* & *B*) Case 2. Right cervical aortic arch. Artist's conception of the anomaly. (From L. W. M. Chang, E. L. Kaplan, D. Baum, and M. M. Figley: Aortic arch in the neck: a case report. *J Pediatr,* 79:788, 1971.)

Case 3. Right cervical aortic arch. At age 2½ years a pulsating mass was detected in the right neck of this child. When the pulsatile mass was occluded, all pulsation except that in the left carotid artery was obliterated. A carotid aneurysm was suspected.

Electrocardiogram was within normal limits. Chest x-ray (Fig. 9-15 *A* & *B*) showed a rather prominent aortic arch and tracheal shift to the left in the cervical region.

Cineangiography and brachial arteriograms (Fig. 9-16) showed a rare anomaly of the aortic arch. The ascending aorta continued to the right into the lower cervical region. At the level of C-7 the aorta made a hairpin loop, crossed obliquely to the left of the vertebral column, and descended in a normal fashion to the left of the spine. The branching of the arch vessels is as shown in Figure 9-17. No treatment for this anomaly was advised. (Courtesy of Dr. William J. Kerth.)

Representative Cases

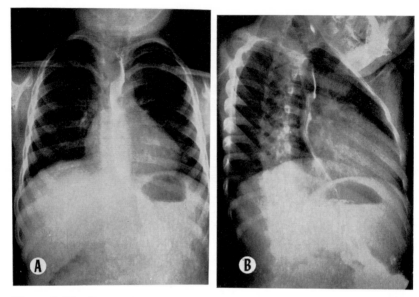

Figure 9-15. Case 3. Right cervical aortic arch. (*A*) A pressure defect in the right upper border of the esophagus at and below the level of the clavicles is evident. The heart is normal. (*B*) Barium swallow in the right anterior oblique projection shows compression of the posterior esophagus at this level. (From R. M. Shepherd, W. J. Kerth, and J. H. Rosenthal: Right cervical aortic arch with left descending aorta. Case report and reveiw of the literature. *Am J Dis Child, 118*:642, 1969.)

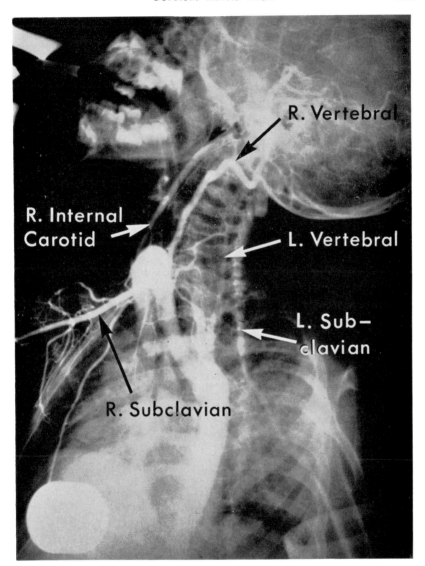

Figure 9-16. Case 3. Right cervical aortic arch. Right brachial arteriogram. Catheter tip lies at the junction of the right subclavian artery and aortic arch. Hairpin turn of the cervical arch is densely opacified. The anatomy of the right cervical aortic arch and the branching of the arch vessels are shown in Figure 9-17. (From R. M. Shepherd, W. J. Kerth, and J. H. Rosenthal: Right cervical aortic arch with left descending aorta. Case report and review of the literature. *Am J Dis Child, 118*:642, 1969.)

Representative Cases

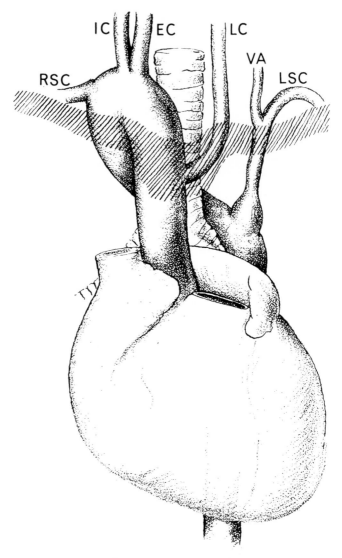

Figure 9-17. Case 3. Right cervical aortic arch. Diagram showing retro-esophageal position of terminal portion of arch, left descending aorta and branching of arch vessels. (From R. M. Shepherd, W. J. Kerth, and J. H. Rosenthal: Right cervical aortic arch with left descending aorta. Case report and review of the literature. *Am J Dis Child, 118*:642, 1969.)

Case 4. Right cervical aortic arch. This seven-year-old boy had stridor of several years duration with frequent respiratory infections. There was a history of a brassy cough present since birth.

Physical examination showed normal blood pressure in both arms and legs. The right carotid and left brachial pulses could not be palpated, and the left axillary pulse was weak. A pulsatile mass protruded from the side of the neck. Electrocardiogram was normal.

Chest roentgenogram (Fig. 9-18) revealed a normal-sized heart. The mediastinal shadow was normal. The aortic knob was not iden-

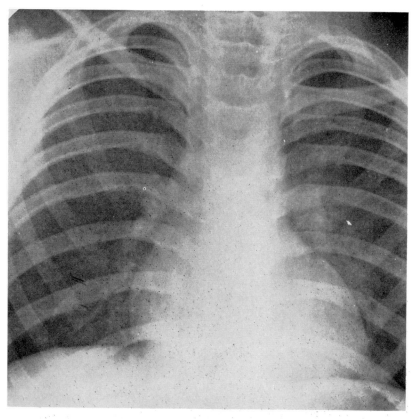

Figure 9-18. Case 4. Right cervical aortic arch. Chest roentgenogram shows a normal mediastinal shadow. The aortic knob is not visible. There is a suggestion of a soft tissue density in the region of the apex of the right lung. (From R. Massumi, L. Wiener, and P. Charif: The syndrome of cervical aorta. Report of a case and review of the previous cases. *Am J Cardiol, 11*:678, 1963.)

Representative Cases

tifiable. The aorta descended on the left. Barium studies (Fig. 9-19 A & B) showed the esophagus to be displaced forward and to the left at the level of T-4.

Aortograms (Fig. 9-20 A & B) revealed a normal ascending aorta. It extended into the neck, crossed the midline behind the esophagus, and descended in normal fashion. The first branch was a large left common carotid artery which originated from the ascending portion. The second branch was a tortuous right subclavian artery arising from the apex of the arch. The right common carotid artery and the origin of the left subclavian artery could not be visualized. Thoracotomy disclosed a vascular ring compressing the trachea and esophagus. An atretic left subclavian artery arose from a conical diverticulum of the aorta just distal to its retroesophageal course. (Courtesy of Dr. Rashid Massumi.)

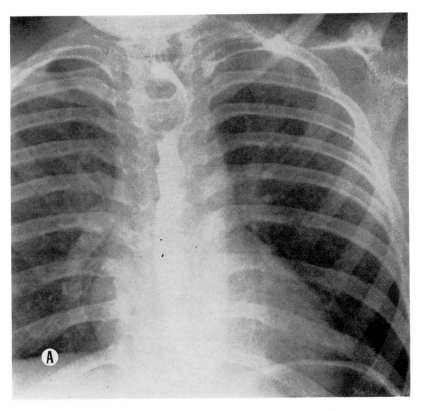

Figure 9-19 A. See legend with Figure 9-19 B.

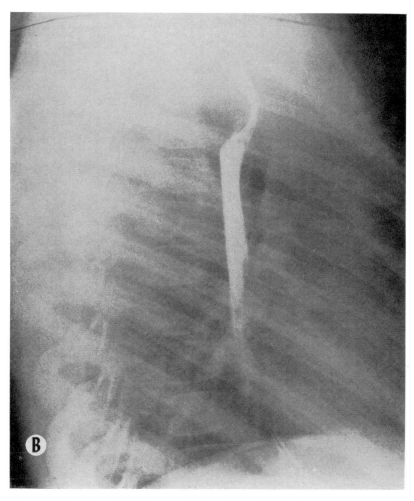

Figure 9-19. Case 4. Right cervical aortic arch. Esophagograms (*A* & *B*) show a localized displacement of the esophagus forward and to the left at the level of the clavicles. (From R. Massumi, L. Wiener, and P. Charif: The syndrome of cervical aorta. Report of a case and review of the previous cases. *Am J Cardiol, 11*:678, 1963.)

Representative Cases

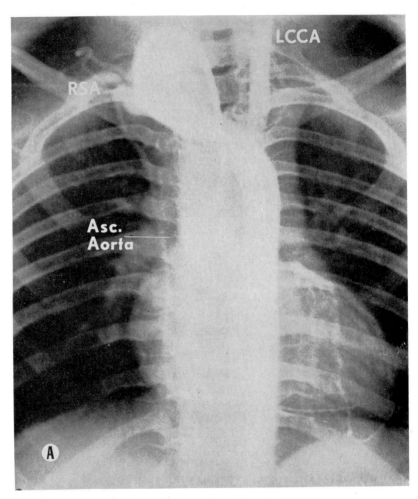

Figure 9-20 A. See legend with 9-20 B.

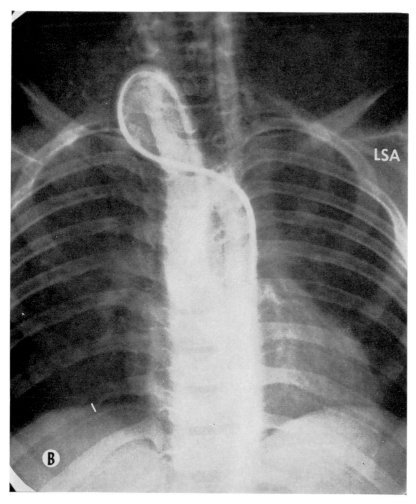

Figure 9-20. Case 4. Right cervical aortic arch. Aortography (*A & B*) shows the aorta to ascend into the right neck, cross the midline and descend on the left side. A large left common carotid artery arises from the ascending aorta as the first branch. (From R. Massumi, L. Wiener, and P. Charif: The syndrome of cervical aorta. Report of a case and review of the previous cases. *Am J Cardiol, 11*:678, 1963.)

Representative Cases

Case 5. Right cervical aortic arch. This ten-year-old girl presented with a large pulsating mass in the right neck. There was no evidence of heart disease nor were there symptoms of a vascular ring.

Retrograde aortograms (Fig. 9-21 *A*, *B*, *C*) showed a very high location of the cervical aorta. The first branch of the right arch was the left common carotid artery. The right internal and external carotid arteries originated independently from the apex of the arch. The origin of the right subclavian artery was from the upper descending portion of the aortic arch. The left subclavian artery arose as the last branch of the arch, from the junction of the retroesophageal and descending portions of the aorta. There appeared to be atresia or severe stenosis of the left subclavian artery near its origin. (Courtesy of Dr. Alois R. Hastreiter.)

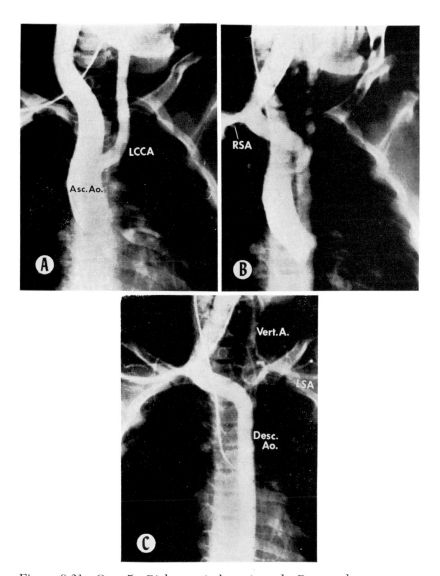

Figure 9-21. Case 5. Right cervical aortic arch. Retrograde aortograms show a very high cervical aortic arch. (*A*) The left common carotid artery arises from the ascending aorta. (*B*) The origin of the right subclavian artery is from the descending portion of the cervical arch. At this point, the aorta crosses the midline to descend on the left side of the spine. (*C*) The left subclavian artery arises as the last branch of the distal arch. Its proximal portion appears to be stenotic, and the left subclavian artery fills by retrograde flow down the vertebral artery. (From A. R. Hastreiter, I. A. D'Cruz, and T. Cantez: Right-sided aorta. *Br Heart J, 28*:722, 1966.)

Representative Cases

Case 6. Right cervical aortic arch. This six-year-old boy presented with a pulsating mass in the right neck. There were no symptoms of tracheal or esophageal compression.

Frontal and lateral levoangiocardiograms are shown in Figure 9-22 A and B. (Courtesy of Dr. Alois R. Hastreiter.)

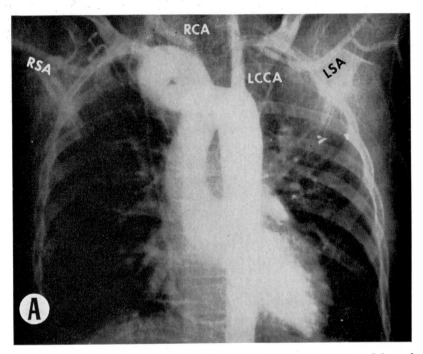

Figure 9-22. Case 6. Right cervical aortic arch. Frontal (A) and lateral (B) levoangiocardiograms shows a normal ascending aorta. It extends into the right supraclavicular region, forms a loop, crosses the midline, to descend on the left side of the spine. The first branch of the right arch is the left common carotid artery, followed by the right carotid arteries, the right subclavian artery, and the left subclavian artery in that order. (From A. R. Hastreiter, I. A. D'Cruz, and T. Cantez: Right-sided aorta. *Br Heart J*, 28:722, 1966.)

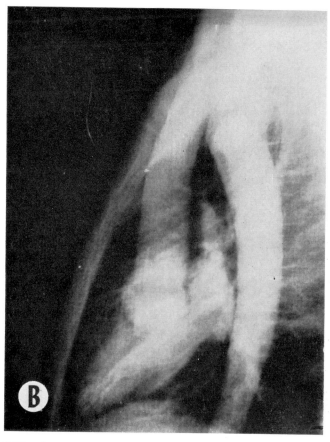

Figure 9-22. Case 6. Right cervical aortic arch. Frontal (*A*) and lateral (*B*) levoangiocardiograms shows a normal ascending aorta. It extends into the right supraclavicular region, forms a loop, crosses the midline, to descend on the left side of the spine. The first branch of the right arch is the left common carotid artery, followed by the right carotid arteries, the right subclavian artery, and the left subclavian artery in that order. (From A. R. Hastreiter, I. A. D'Cruz, and T. Cantez: Right-sided aorta. *Br Heart J*, 28:722, 1966.)

Representative Cases

Case 7. Left cervical aortic arch. This two-year-old boy had repeated respiratory infections which began at three months of age. There was mild stridor and wheezing. He showed findings of tracheal compression with a pulsating mass in the left neck. The roentgen findings are shown in Figure 9-23 *A* and *B*.

Left thoracotomy revealed a high left aortic arch which compressed the trachea and esophagus, but no vascular ring was identified.

At five years of age, an angiocardiogram was performed (Fig. 9-24). Figure 9-25 illustrates the anatomy of the cervical aorta and the branching of the arch vessels. (Courtesy of Dr. Elliott O. Lipchik and Dr. Earle B. Mahoney.)

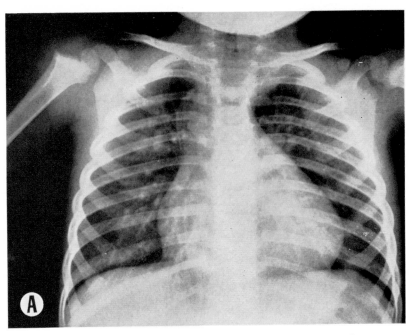

Figure 9-23. Case 7. Left cervical aortic arch. (A) Frontal chest roentgenogram shows a soft tissue shadow to the right of the trachea suggesting a right aortic arch. There is a soft tissue density over the left apex, but no hint of its extension into the left neck. There is slight cardiac enlargement.

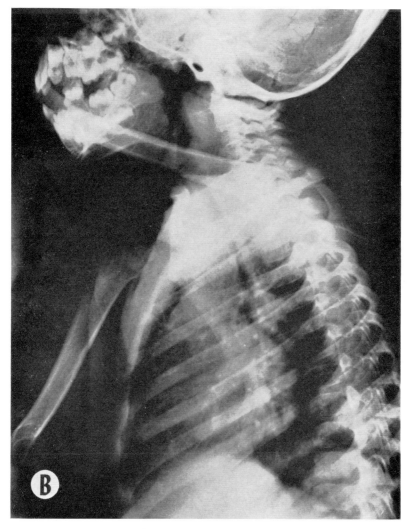

Figure 9-23. Case 7. Left cervical aortic arch. (*B*) Lateral view reveals slight posterior tracheal displacement. (From E. O. Lipchik, and L. W. Young: Unusual symptomatic aortic arch anomalies. *Radiology,* 89:85, 1967.)

Representative Cases

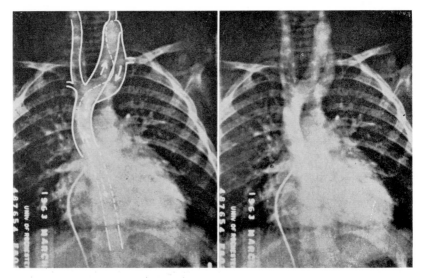

Figure 9-24. Case 7. Left cervical aortic arch. Levoangiocardiogram shows the aorta to ascend on the right with the arch in the left neck. The left common carotid artery arises from the apex of the arch followed by the left subclavian artery. The aorta then crosses the midline to descend on the right. (From E. B. Mahoney, and J. A. Manning: Congenital abnormalities of the aortic arch. *Surgery, 55*:1, 1964.)

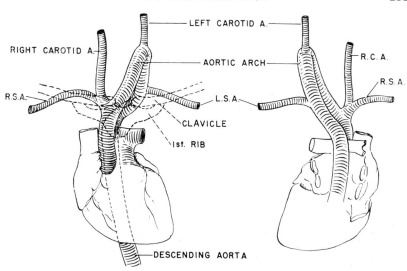

RIGHT CAROTID A.

LEFT CAROTID A.

R.C.A.

AORTIC ARCH

R.S.A.

R.S.A.

L.S.A.

CLAVICLE

1st. RIB

DESCENDING AORTA

CERVICAL LOOP AORTIC ARCH

Figure 9-25. Case 7. Drawing of left cervical aortic arch. (From E. B. Mahoney, and J. A. Manning: Congenital abnormalities of the aortic arch. *Surgery,* 55:1, 1964.)

Case 8. Left cervical aortic arch. This forty-four-year-old woman was asymptomatic except for a pulsatile mass in the left neck. Physical examination showed normal pulsations in the carotid and brachial arteries. The blood pressure was 120/90 mm Hg in both arms.

Chest roentgenogram (Fig. 9-26)revealed a soft tissue mass in the left upper mediastinum extending into the cervical region. The aortic knob could not be identified.

Thoracic aortography (Fig. 9-27 *A* & *B*) showed the left aortic arch extending into the left supraclavicular area and descending on the right side of the thoracic spine. (Courtesy of Dr. Ilse H. de Jong.)

Representative Cases

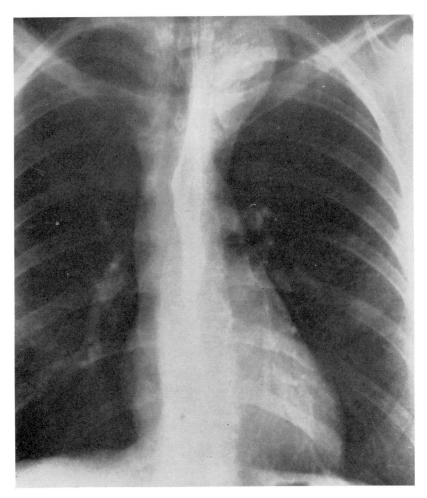

Figure 9-26. Case 8. Left cervical aortic arch. Chest roentgenogram reveals a soft tissue density in the apex of the left lung extending into the cervical region. There is no aortic arch impression on the barium-filled esophagus. (From I. H. de Jong, and A. C. Klinkhamer: Left-sided cervical aortic arch. *Am J Cardiol, 23*:285, 1969.)

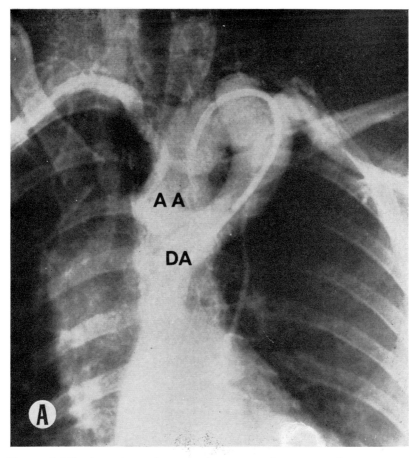

Figure 9-27. Case 8. Left cervical aortic arch. Retrograde aortogram. (A) Frontal view showing the aortic arch high in the left supraclavicular area, with the distal arch crossing the mediastinum, to descend on the right side of the thoracic spine. AA = ascending aorta; DA = descending aorta.

Representative Cases

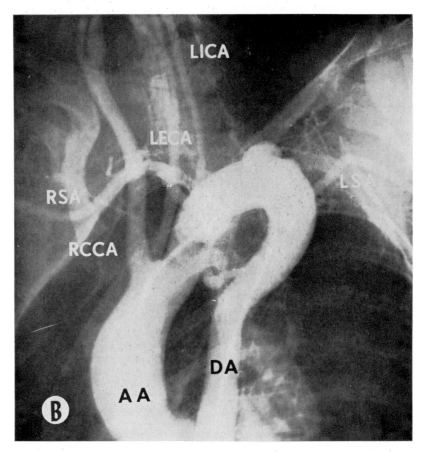

Figure 9-27. Case 8. Left cervical aortic arch. Retrograde aortogram. (*B*) Left anterior oblique view. The first branch of the left arch is the right common carotid artery followed by the left external and internal carotid arteries. The next vessel is the left subclavian artery. The aberrant right subclavian artery arises as the last branch from the distal arch. RCCA = right common carotid artery; LECA = left external carotid artery; LICA = left internal carotid artery; LSA = left subclavian artery; RSA = right subclavian artery. (From I. H. de Jong, and A. C. Klinkhamer: Left-sided cervical aortic arch. *Am J Cardiol*, 23:285, 1969.)

REFERENCES

1. Barry, Alexander: Aortic arch derivatives in the human adult. *Anat Rec, 111*:221, 1951.
2. Beaven, T. E. D., and Fatti, L.: Ligature of aortic arch in the neck. *Br J Surg, 34*:414, 1947.
3. Chang, L. W. M.; Kaplan, E. L.; Baum, D., and Figley, M. M.: Aortic arch in the neck: a case report. *J Pediatr, 79*:788, 1971.
4. Congdon, E. D.: Transformation of the aortic arch system during the development of the human embryo. *Contribut Embryol, 14*:47, 1922.
5. De Jong, I. H., and Klinghamer, A. C.: Left sided cervical aortic arch. *Am J Cardiol, 23*:285, 1969.
6. Edwards, J. E.: Anomalies of the derivatives of the aortic arch system. *Med Clin North Am, 32*:925, 1948.
7. Gravier, J.; Vialtel, M., and Pinet, F.: A propos d'une tumeur pulsatile du con: un cas d'aorte cervieale. *Pediatrie, 437*: 1959.
8. Harley, H. R. S.: The development and anomalies of the aortic arch and its branches. *Br J Surg, 46*:561, 1959.
9. Hastreiter, A. R.; D'Cruz, I. A., and Cantez, T.: Right-sided aorta. *Br Heart J, 28*:722, 1966.
10. Lewis, C., and Rogers, L.: The cervical aortic knuckle which resembles an aneurysm. *Lancet, 1*:825, 1953.
11. Lipchik, Elliot O., and Young, Lionel W.: Unusual symptomatic aortic arch anomalies. *Radiology, 89*:85, 1967.
12. Mahoney, E. B., and Manning, J. A.: Congenital abnormalities of the aortic arch. *Surgery, 55*:1, 1964.
13. Massumi, R.; Wiener, L., and Charif, P.: The syndrome of cervical aorta. Report of a case and review of the previous cases. *Am J Cardiol, 11*:678, 1963.
14. Reid, D. G.: Three examples of a right aortic arch. *J Anat Physiol, 48*:174, 1913.
15. Shepherd, R. M.; Kerth, W. J., and Rosenthal, J. H.: Right cervical aortic arch with left descending aorta. Case report and review of the literature. *Am J Dis Child, 118*:642, 1969.
16. Shuford, W. H.; Sybers, R. G., and Edwards, F. K.: The three types of right aortic arch. *Am J Roentgenol Radium Ther Nucl Med, 109*:67, 1970.
17. Shuford, W. H.; Sybers, R. G., and Weens, H. S.: The angiographic features of double aortic arch. *Am J Roentgenol Radium Ther Nucl Med, 116*:125, 1972.
18. Shuford, W. H.; Sybers, R. G.; Milledge, R. D., and Brinsfield, D.: The cervical aortic arch. *Am J Roentgenol Radium Ther Nucl Med, 116*:519, 1972.

19. Stewart, J. R.; Kincaid, O. W., and Edwards, J. E.: *An Atlas of Vascular Rings and Related Malformations of the Aortic Arch System.* Thomas, Springfield, 1964, pp. 8-13, 124-129.

CHAPTER 10

INTERRUPTION OF THE AORTIC ARCH

Definition. Two forms of interruption of the aortic arch are recognized. In one form, there is complete anatomic interruption of the arch. In the other, an atretic fibrous remnant connects the proximal arch with the descending aorta.[1, 3] This latter type has been referred to as atresia of the aortic arch.[4] In this section, we are limiting our discussion to these cases of interruption of the aortic arch in which there is no anatomic connection between the proximal aorta and descending portion. Atresia of the aortic arch is discussed in the following section.

A patent ductus arteriosus is present and provides the circulatory pathway to the descending aorta.[4] Multiple anatomic variations are possible depending upon the sites of origin of the brachiocephalic vessels.[1]

Incidence and Clinical Significance. This is an uncommon malformation of the aortic arch. We have performed angiographic studies on one patient with this condition in which a truncus arteriosus was also present. In about one half of the reported cases, the brachiocephalic vessels originated from the proximal aorta. In approximately one third of the reported cases, the left subclavian artery arose from the descending aorta, and the left common carotid and the innominate artery arose from the ascending aorta.[1] Interruption of the aortic arch with the right and left subclavian arteries arising from the descending aorta and the right and left common carotid arteries originating from the proximal aorta account for 10 percent of the reported cases.[1] Other variations in branching of the arch vessels are rarely encountered.

189

This anomaly is one of the causes of the hypoplastic left heart syndrome.[3] Most infants with this malformation have congestive heart failure early in life.[3] Almost always a ventricular septal defect is present, either as an isolated intracardiac defect (approximately 50 percent of cases) or part of a more severe cardiac malformation, such as subaortic stenosis, complete transposition of the great arteries, truncus arteriosus or right ventricular origin of both great vessels. Less than 5 percent of cases have no intracardiac anomaly.[1, 3]

Development. Interruption of the aortic arch results from a complete break in both the right and left embryonic arches in the hypothetical double aortic arch system.

Most often interruption occurs distal to the subclavian artery in the double aortic arch (Fig. 10-1). In the embryonic left arch interruption is between the left subclavian artery and the left ductus arteriosus. In the embryonic right arch interruption is between the right subclavian artery and descending aorta. In this variation, all the barchiocephalic vessels arise from the proximal aorta. About one half of all cases of interruption of the aortic arch have this type of development.

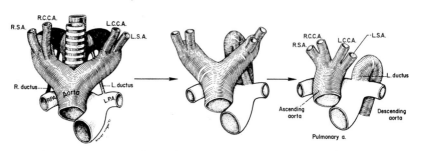

Figure 10-1. Development of interruption of the aortic arch with each brachiocephalic artery arising from the proximal aorta. Areas in black indicate segments of complete regression of each embryonic arch in the hypothetical double aortic arch.

Or interruption may take place between the left common carotid and left subclavian arteries in the embryonic left arch, and between the right subclavian artery and descending aorta in the embryonic right arch (Fig. 10-2). In this pattern, the left subclavian artery arises from the descending aorta, and the left common carotid artery and the innominate artery arise from the proximal aorta. In approximately one third of all reported cases of interruption of the aortic arch the branching of the arch vessels is of this type.

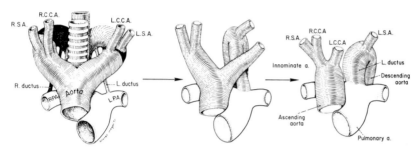

Figure 10-2. Development of interruption of the aortic arch with the left subclavian artery arising from the descending aorta. The innominate artery and the left common carotid artery originate from the ascending aorta. Areas in black indicate segments of complete regression of each embryonic arch in the hypothetical double aortic arch.

Less often, interruption occurs between the common carotid and subclavian arteries in both embryonic aortic arches (Fig. 10-3). In this variation, the right and left subclavian arteries arise from the descending aorta and the right and left common carotid arteries originate from the proximal aorta. Approximately 10 percent of cases of interruption of the aortic arch have this branching of the arch vessels.

Interruption at other sites has been reported, but these cases are quite uncommon.

Chest Roentgenography. The chest x-ray shows considerable cardiac enlargement, especially when congestive heart failure is present. There is usually increased pulmonary arterial vasculature.

In most cases, barium studies of the esophagus revealed no abnormality. In approximately 10 percent of patients with interruption of the aortic arch, the right subclavian artery arises from the descending aorta.[1] In these patients, the esophagogram may show an oblique filling defect on the frontal view and a posterior

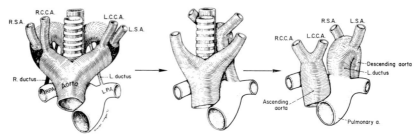

Figure 10-3. Development of interruption of the aortic arch with the right common carotid artery and the left common carotid artery arising from the proximal aorta and the right subclavian artery and the left subclavian artery arising from the descending aorta. Areas in black indicate segments of complete regression of each embryonic arch in the hypothetical double aortic arch.

compression defect on the lateral projection at the level of the aorta arch.

Angiographic Features. Selective angiography and aortography demonstrate the sites of origin of the brachiocephalic vessels. A large patent ductus arteriosus is the most constant feature and provides the circulatory pathway to the descending aorta.[3] The associated cardiac malformation may be demonstrated.

Representative Case

Case 1. Interruption of aortic arch with both subclavian arteries arising from the descending aorta and the common carotid arteries arising from the proximal aorta with persistent truncus arteriosus.

This 3000 gram infant was noted to have a loud heart murmur on her initial physical examination. On the second day of life, congestive heart failure and cyanosis developed. Physical examination showed mild cyanosis. Blood pressures were 58/30 mm Hg in the right arm and 66/40 mm Hg in the left arm. The heart was enlarged with a systolic thrill along the left sternal border. A systolic murmur was heard over the anterior chest and seemed to be continuous at the right upper sternal border.

Electrocardiogram showed biventricular hypertrophy. Chest x-ray revealed marked cardiomegaly and increased pulmonary blood flow (Fig. 10-4).

Selective right ventricular angiocardiography showed filling of a large pulmonary trunk followed by immediate opacification of what appeared to be the ascending aorta. The descending aorta opacified through a large ductus arteriosus (Fig. 10-5 A & B). Left retrograde brachial arteriography (Fig. 10-6 *A* & *B*) showed simultaneous opacification of the pulmonary trunk and the proximal aorta as well as descending aorta. The proximal aorta gave rise to the right and left common carotid arteries and was interrupted at this point. The right and left subclavian arteries arose from the proximal descending aorta. There was regurgitation of contrast material into the ventricles.

A diagnosis of persistent truncus arteriosus with interruption of the aortic arch distal to the left common carotid artery with the right subclavian artery originating from the descending aorta and insufficiency of the truncal valve was made.

Figure 10-7 is a diagram of the anomalies found at postmortem examination. The heart was greatly enlarged with a large defect in the membranous portion of the ventricular septum. A short pulmonary trunk arose directly from the truncus arteriosus and gave rise to the right and left pulmonary arterial branches. The three truncal valve cusps were thickened, deformed and incompetent. There was complete interruption of the aortic arch distal to the left common carotid artery. The right subclavian artery had an aberrant origin from the proximal descending aorta passing behind the esophagus to reach the right arm. A large patent ductus arteriosus connected the pulmonary artery to the descending aorta.

Representative Cases

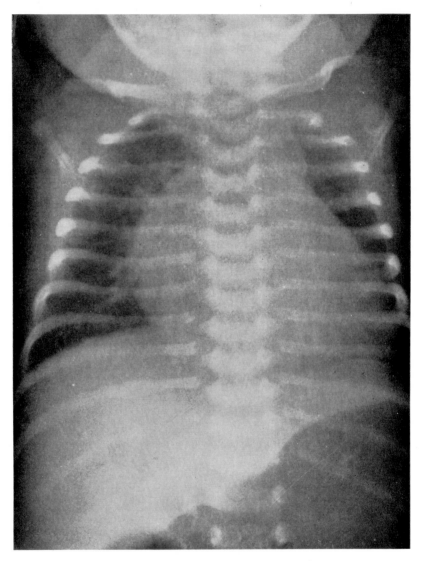

Figure 10-4. Case 1. Interruption of aortic arch. Chest roentgenogram shows generalized cardiomegaly and increased pulmonary vasculature.

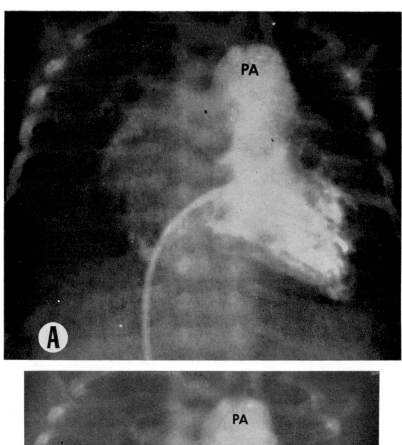

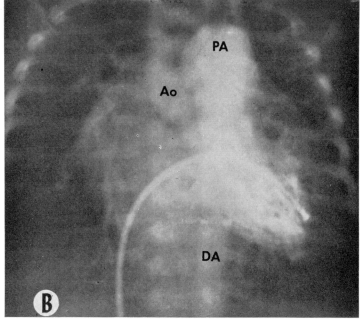

Figure 10-5. Case 1. Interruption of aortic arch. Selective right ventricular angiocardiogram. (A) There is filling of a large pulmonary trunk. (B) One second later, there is opacification of the proximal aorta. The descending aorta opacifies via a large ductus arteriosus.

Representative Cases

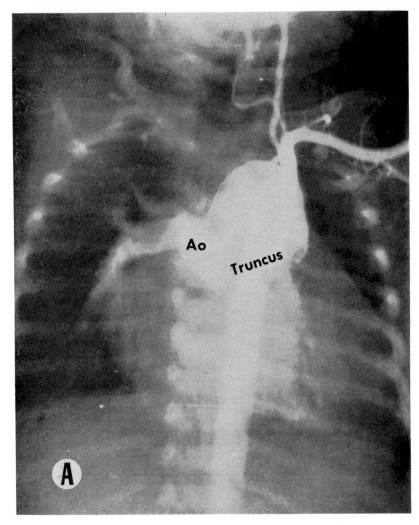

Figure 10-6. Case 1. Interruption of aortic arch. Retrograde countercurrent left brachial arteriogram. (A) Contrast material passes retrograde from left subclavian artery with simultaneous filling of the proximal aorta, pulmonary trunk and descending aorta.

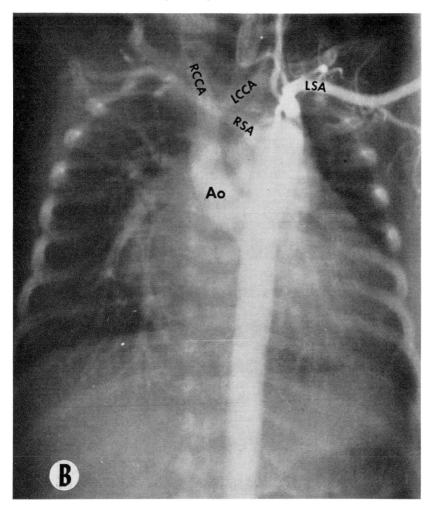

Figure 10-6. Case 1. Interruption of aortic arch. Retrograde countercurrent left brachial arteriogram. (*B*) The proximal aorta is interrupted and gives rise to the right and left common carotid arteries. The right and left subclavian arteries originate from the descending aorta.

Representative Cases

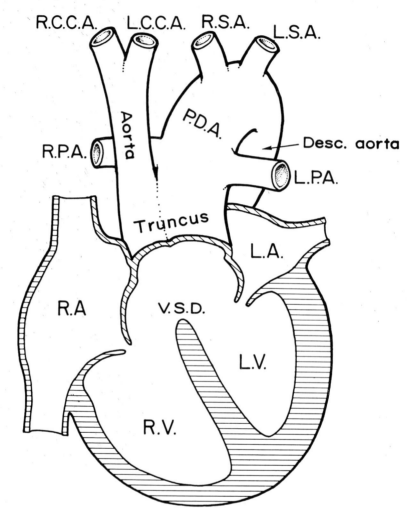

Figure 10-7. Case 1. Interruption of aortic arch. Diagram of cardiac anatomy. Both ventricles empty into a truncus arteriosus through a membranous ventricular septal defect. A short pulmonary trunk arises directly from the truncus. There is complete interruption of the aortic arch distal to the left common carotid artery. The right subclavian artery arises from the descending aorta and passes behind the esophagus to reach the right arm. A large patent ductus provides the circulatory pathway from the main pulmonary artery to the descending aorta.

Atresia of the Aortic Arch

Definition. In this malformation an atretic fibrous remnant without a lumen connects the ascending aorta with the descending aorta. A physiological interruption of the aortic arch results.[3] It is for this reason that most authors have included this condition under the designation of interruption of the aortic arch. Direct inspection is necessary to distinguish atresia of the aortic arch from true anatomic interruption.

A patent ductus arteriosus is present, and the ascending aorta is supplied by the left ventricle, and the descending aorta by the right ventricle through the ductus arteriosus.[4]

Incidence and Clinical Significance. Atresia of the aortic arch is uncommon. A few of the reported cases of interruption of the aortic arch represent true examples of aortic arch atresia.[1]

Obstruction to blood flow through the hypoplastic left heart is the fundamental circulatory disturbance.[3] Severe congestive heart failure, usually within the first few days of life, is the principal finding. This malformation is usually part of a complicated cardiac anomaly.

Development. Atresia of the aortic arch results from complete regression of the right embryonic arch and partial regression of the left embryonic arch in the hypothetical double aortic arch system. In the most common form, all the brachiocephalic vessels arise from the proximal aorta. Figure 10-8 shows the development of this variation.

In the next common form, the left subclavian artery arises from the descending aorta and the left common carotid artery and the innominate artery arise from the proximal aorta.[1] This pattern develops from complete interruption of the right embryonic arch distal to the right subclavian artery and partial regression of the left embryonic arch between the left common carotid and left subclavian arteries. Less often, complete interruption of the right arch between the right common carotid and right subclavian arteries and partial regression of the left arch between the left common carotid and left subclavian arteries takes place.

Chest Roentgenography. The chest roentgenogram reflects

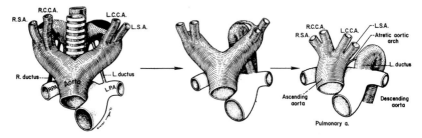

Figure 10-8. Development of atresia of the aortic arch with the atretic segment distal to the left subclavian artery. Each brachiocephalic vessel arises from the ascending aorta proximal to the site of atresia. There has been complete regression of the right embryonic arch distal to the right subclavian artery and partial regression of the left embryonic arch beyond the left subclavian artery.

the severe congestive heart failure that is present. Cardiomegaly is usually marked.

Angiographic Features. The left ventricle supplies the ascending aorta and the descending aorta is supplied by the right ventricle through the patent ductus. The origins of the brachiocephalic vessels are usually demonstrated.

Representative Case

Case 2. Atresia of aortic arch with the brachiocephalic vessels arising from the proximal aorta and truncus arteriosus. This 3200 gram male was noted at the age of three days to have symptoms and signs of congestive heart failure. A loud continuous murmur, more ejection in type at the cardiac base, was present along the left sternal border. A systolic thrill was palpable along the left sternal border and transmitted to the left neck. Blood pressure was 70/40 mm Hg in both arms and 75/35 mm Hg in the right leg.

The electrocardiogram showed findings of biventricular hypertrophy. Chest roentgenogram (Fig. 10-9) revealed generalized cardiomegaly and pulmonary plethora. The clinical impression was persistent truncus arteriosus with congestive heart failure.

Selective right ventrciular angiocardiography (Fig. 10-10 A & B) demonstrated a ventricular septal defect and simultaneous filling of the pulmonary arteries and brachiocephalic vessels. The descending aorta appeared to fill from the pulmonary trunk via the ductus arteriosus. Retrograde aortography (Fig. 10-11) showed a truncus arteriosus with complete interruption of the aortic arch distal to the left subclavian artery and mild insufficiency of the truncal valve. The descending aorta filled from the ductus. The infant died at six days of age.

Postmortem examination revealed a greatly enlarged heart with a single vessel arising from the base of the heart overriding a membranous ventricular septal defect. This vessel had four valve cusps which appeared thickened and fibrotic. The main pulmonary artery arose from the truncus 9 mm above the valve and divided into a right and left branch. The ascending aorta supplied the brachio-

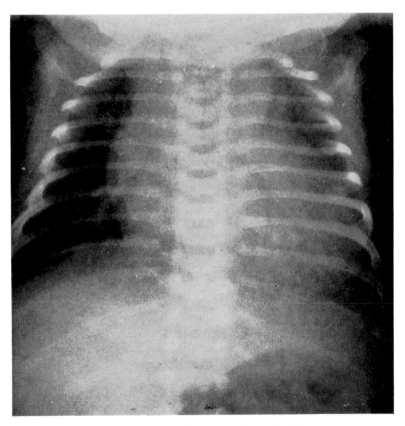

Figure 10-9. Case 2. Atresia of the aortic arch. Chest roentgenogram shows marked cardiomegaly and increased pulmonary vasculature. (From A. D. Morgan, D. Brinsfield, and F. K. Edwards: Persistent truncus arteriosus—an unusual variant with atresia of the aortic arch. *Am J Dis Child*, 109:74, 1965.)

cephalic vessels before becoming atretic. A small fibrotic strand connected the aortic arch with the ductus arteriosus and descending
aorta (Fig. 10-12). Two coronary arteries arose from the base of
the truncus. (Courtesy of Dr. Dorothy Brinsfield and Dr. Kathryn
Edwards.)

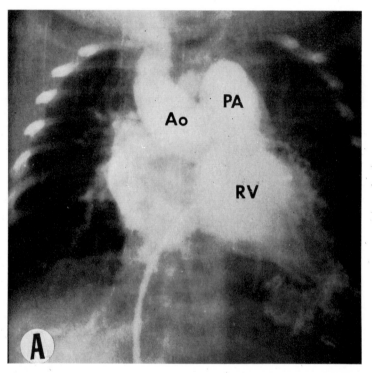

Figure 10-10. Case 2. Atresia of the aortic arch. Right ventriculogram
(A) shows simultaneous filling of the brachiocephalic vessels and pulmonary arteries with interruption of the aortic arch distal to the left subclavian artery.

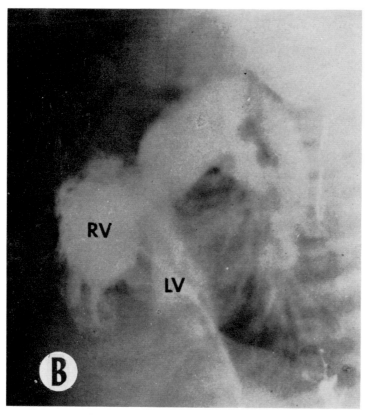

Figure 10-10. Case 2. Atresia of the aortic arch. Lateral view (*B*) reveals contrast material passing from the right to the left ventricle through a ventricular septal defect. (From A. D. Morgan, D. Brinsfield, and F. K. Edwards: Persistent truncus arteriosus—an unusual variant with atresia of the aortic arch. *Am J Dis Child, 109*:74, 1965.)

Representative Cases

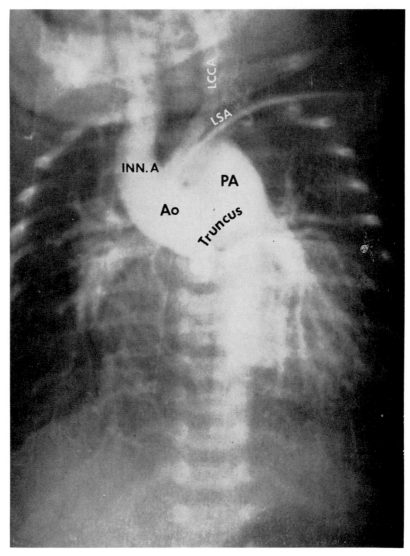

Figure 10-11. Case 2. Atresia of the aortic arch. Aortogram (catheter introduced via left brachial artery with injection of opaque material into proximal aorta). The truncus, brachiocephalic vessels, pulmonary vessels and descending aorta are filled. There is regurgitation of contrast material into both ventricles. (From A. D. Morgan, D. Brinsfield, and F. K. Edwards: Persistent truncus arteriosus—an unusual variant with atresia of the aortic arch. *Am J Dis Child, 109*:74, 1965.)

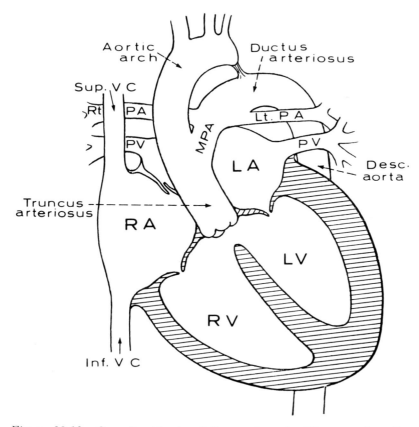

Figure 10-12. Case 2. Atresia of the aortic arch. Diagram of cardiac anatomy. The truncus arteriosus overrides a membranous ventricular septal defect. The main pulmonary artery arises from the truncus and divides into a right and left branch. The proximal aorta gives rise to the brachiocephalic vessels and becomes atretic distal to the left subclavian artery. A fibrotic strand connects the aortic arch with the descending aorta. A large patent ductus arteriosus provides the circulatory pathway from the main pulmonary artery to the descending aorta. (From A. D. Morgan, D. Brinsfield, and F. K. Edwards: Persistent truncus arteriosus—an unusual variant with atresia of the aortic arch. *Am J Dis Child,* 109:74, 1965.)

REFERENCES

1. Moller, J. H., and Edwards, J. E.: Interruption of the aortic arch anatomic patterns and associated cardiac malformations. *Am J Roentgenol Radium Ther Nucl Med, 95*:557, 1965.
2. Morgan, A. D.; Brinsfield, D., and Edwards, F. K.: Persistent truncus arteriosus. *Am J Dis Child, 109*:74, 1965.
3. Perloff, J. K.: *The Clinical Recognition of Congenital Heart Disease.* Philadelphia, Saunders, 1970, pp. 586-588.
4. Roberts, W. C.; Morrow, A. G., and Braunwald, E.: Complete interruption of the aortic arch. *Circulation, 26*:39, 1962.

CHAPTER 11

HYPOPLASTIC CONDITIONS OF THE AORTA

IN THIS CHAPTER we will consider some conditions in which a portion of the ascending aorta or aortic arch is hypoplastic. The term hypoplasia of the aorta as used here refers to a state of arrested development in which the lumen of the aorta is narrowed but patent, and the size of the vessel is diminished. While hypoplasia of the aorta may be localized, generally a rather long segment of the aorta is involved. The conditions discussed here are (a) *aortic valve atresia*, (b) *coarctation of the aorta* and (c) *supravalvular aortic stenosis*.

Aortic Valve Atresia

Definition. Aortic atresia is characterized by complete closure of the aortic orifice.[4, 6, 10] There is marked underdevelopment of the left side of the heart. The ascending aorta is always patent. Usually the ascending aorta is hypoplastic, although on rare occasions it may be of essentially normal caliber.[9] The right ventricle supplies the entire pulmonary and systemic circulation.[10] A widely patent ductus arteriosus delivers blood to the aorta.[10] From this source, blood flows retrograde into the proximal aorta to supply the coronary arteries.

Incidence and Clinical Significance. Congenital atresia of the aortic valve is not a rare anomaly. It is one of the most common causes of death from congenital heart disease within the first week of life.[4] Infants with this anomaly may appear normal at birth, but they quickly develop severe congestive heart failure during the first and second days of life.[10]

Development. Complete closure of the aortic orifice results in marked underdevelopment (hypoplasia) of the ascending aorta.[2]

Chest Roentgenography. The heart shadow may be normal at birth. However, there is usually cardiac enlargement due to dilatation of the right atrium, right ventricle and pulmonary trunk. The hilar shadows are congested.[6]

Angiographic Features. Opacification of the right side of the heart reveals a large right atrium and right ventricle. From the pulmonary artery, a large patent ductus arteriosus supplies blood to the aorta, opacifying the arch and descending aorta.

Retrograde aortogram reveals the hypoplastic ascending aorta filling in retrograde fashion to supply the coronary arteries.

Representative Cases

Case 1. Aortic valve atresia. This term male infant developed heart failure at two days of age.

Chest roentgenograms showed cardiac enlargement. The right heart border was particularly prominent. The lungs were markedly congested.

Angiocardiography (Fig. 11-1 *A* & *B*) revealed opacification of the pulmonary artery and descending aorta simultaneously. The right side of the heart was dilated, and the main pulmonary artery was enlarged. Countercurrent left brachial arteriography (Fig. 11-2 *A* & *B*) demonstrated retrograde flow down a severely under-developed ascending aorta which supplied the coronary arteries. There was an abrupt cutoff of the opacified aortic arch where the ductus arteriosus delivered nonopacified blood into the aorta.

Postmortem examination demonstrated aortic valve atresia. The ascending aorta was hypoplastic. The mitral valve was hypoplastic, but structurally was normal and was associated with a small ventricular cavity. The foramen ovale was patent.

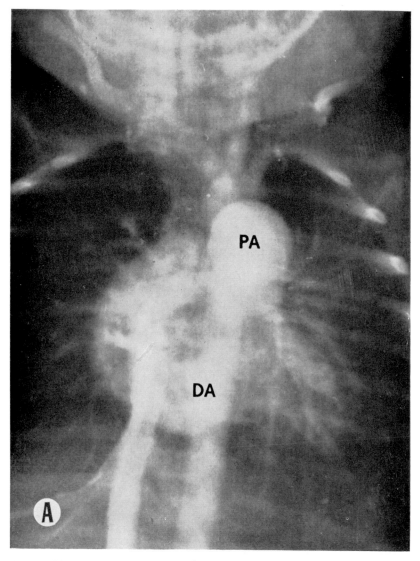

Figure 11-1. Case 1. Aortic valve atresia. Frontal (A) venous angio-cardiogram shows enlarged right atrium, right ventricle and pulmonary artery. There is simultaneous opacification of the aortic arch and descending aorta via a large patent ductus arteriosus.

Representative Cases

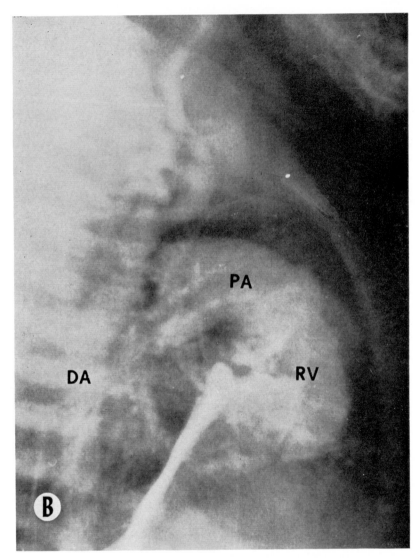

Figure 11-1. Case 1. Aortic valve atresia. Lateral (*B*) venous angio-cardiogram shows enlarged right atrium, right ventricle and pulmonary artery. There is simultaneous opacification of the aortic arch and descending aorta via a large patent ductus arteriosus.

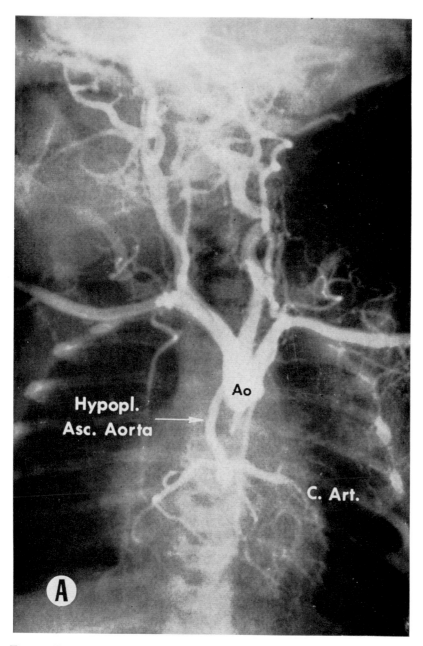

Figure 11-2. Case 1. Aortic valve atresia. Frontal (A) retrograde countercurrent brachial arteriogram shows a severely hypoplastic aorta with retrograde filling of the coronary arteries. The branching of the arch vessels is normal. There is an abrupt cutoff of the opacified aortic arch where the large patent ductus arteriosus delivers nonopaque blood to the aorta.

Representative Cases

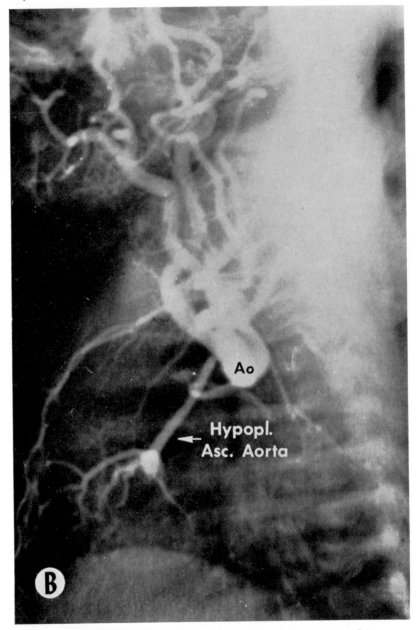

Figure 11-2. Case 1. Aortic valve atresia. Lateral (*B*) retrograde counter-current brachial arteriogram shows a severely hypoplastic aorta with retrograde filling of the coronary arteries.

Case 2. Aortic valve atresia. Term infant with dyspnea, cyanosis, marked tachycardia, enlarged liver, enormously enlarged heart. Retrograde aortogram (Fig. 11-3) showed a markedly hypoplastic ascending aorta.

Representative Cases

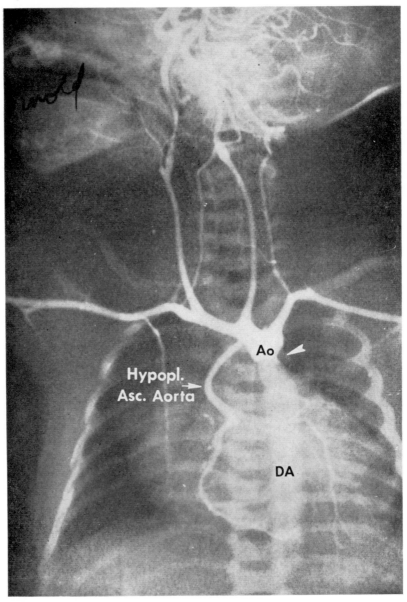

Figure 11-3. Case 2. Aortic valve atresia. Retrograde countercurrent brachial arteriogram showing hypoplastic ascending aorta. The descending aorta below where the patent ductus delivers nonopaque blood to the aorta (arrow) is considerably less opacified than the aortic arch.

Coarctation of the Aorta

Definition. The essential feature of this malformation is a localized deformity of the aortic media resulting in a curtain-like infolding of the wall which causes an eccentric narrowing of the aortic lumen—hence the term coarctation which refers to a condition of stricture or contracture.[10] Coarctation most often occurs at the beginning of the descending thoracic aorta distal to the left subclavian artery at, or near, the insertion of the ductus arteriosus.[4] On rare occasions, the aortic coarctation may be proximal to the origin of the left subclavian artery.[1, 2, 8, 13]

Coarctation may be the only aortic narrowing present, the remainder of the aorta being of normal size with preservation of a normal lumen. Usually, however, a zone of hypoplasia is present. Hypoplasia, as used here, refers to a segment of aorta with a narrowed lumen in which the media is histologically normal.[4]

Most commonly, the hypoplastic segment involves the isthmus of the aorta (that portion between the left subclavian artery and ductus arteriosus).[7] The caliber of this hypoplastic zone is frequently of the same size as the left subclavian artery. In other patients, the hypoplasia not only involves the isthmus, but extends further into the aortic arch.

The relationship of the aortic insertion of the ductus arteriosus to the coarctate segment may explain the development of the aortic hypoplasia.[4, 10] Figure 11-4 shows a tight aortic coarctation with the ductus entering the aorta distal to the coarctation. Under these circumstances, blood flow during fetal life is from the right ventricle through the ductus arteriosus to the descending aorta. Ductal flow cannot reach the proximal aorta. Thus, flow in the ascending aorta and aortic arch is diminished, and the aortic arch and isthmus may show varying degrees of underdevelopment.

When the ductus arteriosus enters the aorta proximal to the site of coarctation (Fig. 11-5), the entire systemic and pulmonary circulations are directed to the aortic arch and blood reaches the descending thoracic aorta via collateral pathways. There is no diminution of blood flow in the ascending aorta and arch, and in these patients one would not expect to see hypopolasia of the arch.

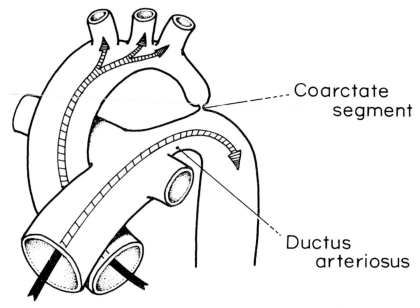

Figure 11-4. Severe coarctation of the aorta proximal to the ductus arteriosus. Fetal blood flow is from the right ventricle through the ductus to the descending aorta. Ductal flow is not directed to the aortic arch. There is diminution of blood flow in the aortic arch and isthmus which are hypoplastic.

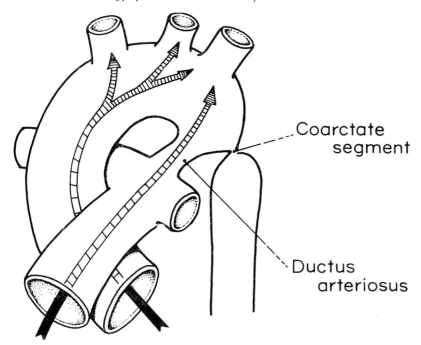

Figure 11-5. Severe coarctation of the aorta distal to ductus arteriosus. The entire systemic and pulmonary circulations are directed to the aortic arch. There is no diminution of blood flow in the ascending aorta and arch. The aortic arch is not hypoplastic.

Incidence and Clinical Significance. Coarctation of the aorta is twice as common in males as in females.[6] Children over one year of age with coarctation of the aorta usually have no symptoms, and the defect is discovered during examinaion for some other reason.[10] Usually, these patients are examined because of a heart murmur or hypertension.

Approximately one half of patients with coarctation discovered in childhood will have symptoms in the first year of life.[6] Severe congestive heart failure may occur with no other lesions. However, the majority of infants with symptoms have associated cardiac defects.[4]

In some patients there may be an associated aberrant right subclavian artery, arising as the most distal branch of the aortic arch.[5, 7, 12] Rib notching in coarctation may provide information regarding the location of the coarctate segment in relation to the origin of the aberrant subclavian vessel.[3] If the origin of the aberrant right subclavian artery is distal to the site of coarctation, or is stenotic, the right subclavian artery is a low pressure artery, and rib notching occurs on the left side only.[5] If the origin of the aberrant right subclavian artery is proximal to the coarctation, both arms are hypertensive and rib notching may be present on both sides.[3]

When the aortic coarctation is proximal to the left subclavian artery, rib notching occurs on the right side only, unless there is also associated anomalous origin of the right subclavian artery distal to the coarctation.[1, 2, 8, 13] In these patients, rib notching should not develop on either side.

Chest Roentgenography. In the symptomatic infant, the chest roentgenogram reveals findings of congestive heart failure with marked cardiac enlargement and left atrial preponderance.[6] The lung fields are congested. The pulmonary blood flow is normal in the absence of associated cardiac defects.

Patients over one year of age usually show no cardiac enlargement.[10] Notching of the ribs may be present, although rib notching is rarely encountered before the age of ten years.[3] There may be a dilated ascending aorta or evidence of a hypoplastic arch. Post-stenotic dilatation of the aorta may be a conspicuous feature.

Angiographic Features. Retrograde aortography will readily show the site of coarctation and the hypoplastic segment. If the ductus arteriosus is patent, flow from the aorta to the pulmonary artery may be visualized. In most patients, particularly adults, the collateral circulation is visible.

In patients with coarctation of the aorta in whom the right subclavian artery has an aberrant origin from the aortic arch, blood flow in the aberrant subclavian vessel is determined by the origin of the aberrant vessel in relation to the coarctate segment.[4] If the aberrant right subclavian artery arises proximal to the aortic coarctation, blood flow in the right subclavian artery will be in the usual direction (Fig. 11-10). If the aberrant right subclavian artery arises distal to the aortic coarctation, blood flow is in retrograde fashion and provides a large collateral pathway to the lower pressure descending aorta.[5,12] Under these circumstances, there is retrograde flow down the right vertebral artery to fill the right subclavian artery and subsequently the descending thoracic aorta distal to the coarctation (right-sided subclavian steal syndrome) (Fig. 11-11 A-D; Fig. 11-12 A, B, C; Fig. 11-13). These pathways of collateral circulation are illustrated in Figure 5-35.

Representative Cases

Case 3. Coarctation of the aorta. This infant was hospitalized at twelve days of age with severe congestive heart failure which responded well to medical therapy.

Aortographic studies (Fig. 11-6 A & B) revealed coarctation of the aorta with narrowing just distal to the left subclavian artery with an opening measuring approximately two to three millimeters.

At age seven years, the child was admitted to the hospital for resection of the aortic coarctation. Blood pressure in both arms was 150/110 mm Hg and the blood pressure in the legs was unobtainable. The pulses in the legs could not be felt.

At surgery, there was a very tight juxtaductal coarctation with marked dilatation of the left subclavian artery and left internal mammary artery as well as the intercostal arteries. The coarctate segment was excised and an end-to-end anastamosis was performed.

Representative Cases

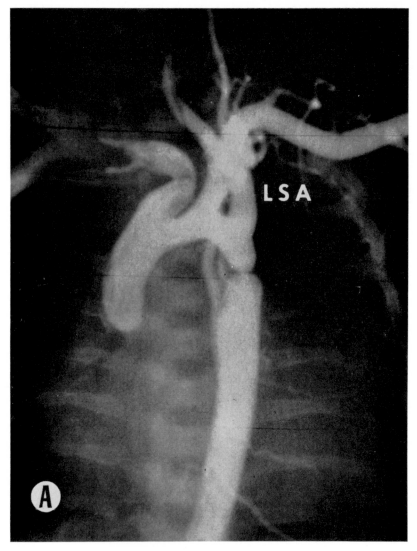

Figure 11-6. Case 3. Coarctation of the aorta. Frontal (A) aortogram shows a localized juxtaductal coarctation well beyond the origin of the left subclavian artery. There is post-stenotic dilatation beyond the narrow segment. The internal mammary artery is enlarged, feeding the intercostal arteries as collateral channels to the descending aorta.

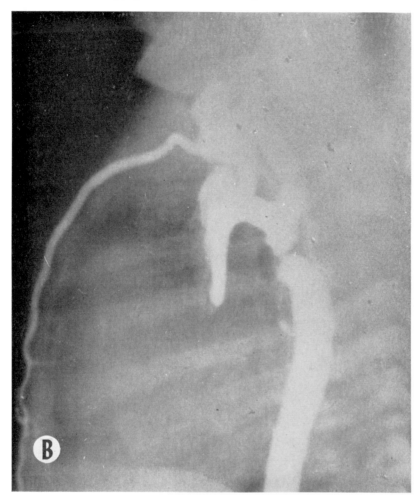

Figure 11-6. Case 3. Coarctation of the aorta. Lateral (*B*) aortogram shows a localized juxtaductal coarctation well beyond the origin of the left subclavian artery. There is post-stenotic dilatation beyond the narrow segment. The internal mammary artery is enlarged, feeding the intercostal arteries as collateral channels to the descending aorta.

Representative Cases

Case 4. Coarctation of the aorta. This twelve-year-old child was referred to the cardiac clinic because of a heart murmur which was heard on routine examination. She gave a history of mild exertional dyspnea and some cramping in the legs with exercise.

Physical examination revealed a grade III systolic murmur in the pulmonic area radiating along the left sternal border. A systolic murmur was also audible in the back. The carotid pulses were bounding and the radial pulses were prominent. No pulses were palpable in the lower extremities. Blood pressure in both arms was 150/80 mm Hg and it was impossible to obtain blood pressures in the legs by auscultation.

Aortography (Fig. 11-7 A & B) disclosed a localized site of coarctation distal to the left subclavian artery with post-stenotic dilatation of the descending aorta. The arch vessels were dilated. There was a zone of hypoplasia involving the aortic isthmus.

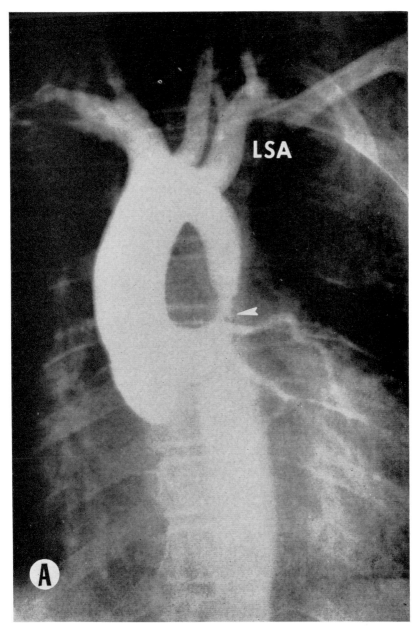

Figure 11-7. Case 4. Coarctation of the aorta. Retrograde aortograms. (A) Arrow points to coarctate segment. The aortic isthmus is hypoplastic. Post-stenotic dilatation of the aorta is marked.

Representative Cases

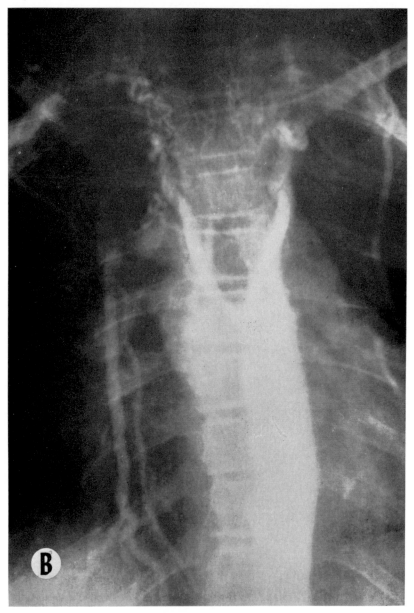

Figure 11-7. Case 4. Coarctation of the aorta. Retrograde aortogram.
(*B*) Both internal mammary arteries are dilated and provide a collateral
pathway to the descending aorta.

Case 5. Coarctation of the aorta. This thirteen-day-old male infant four days prior to admission developed vomiting and grunting respirations with deep breathing.

Physical examination revealed cardiomegaly with rapid respirations. The liver was enlarged. The radial pulses were more easily palpable than the femoral pulses.

Shortly after admission, aortography (Fig. 11-8 *A* & *B*) revealed a localized severe coarctation of the aorta distal to the left subclavian artery with a zone of hypoplasia of the aortic arch. There was opacification of the pulmonary artery through a large patent ductus arteriosus just distal to the aortic coarctation. The upper descending aorta showed post-stenotic dilatation. Several hours after the examination, the child expired.

Representative Cases

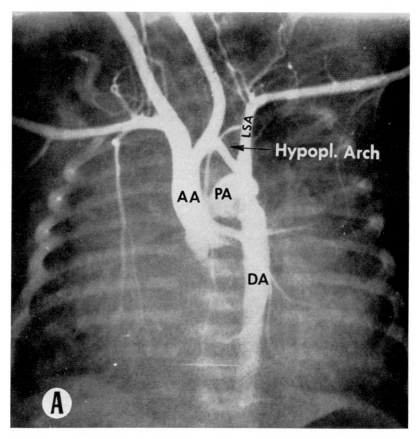

Figure 11-8. Case 5. Coarctation of the aorta. Frontal (A) retrograde aortogram. (A) There is a marked decrease in the caliber of the aortic lumen extending from a point just distal to the origin of the left common carotid artery past the origin of the left subclavian artery.

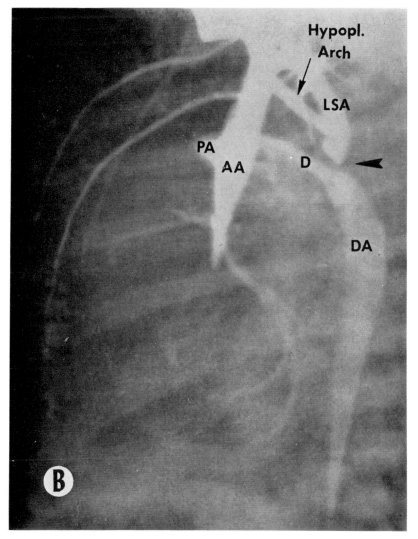

Figure 11-8. Case 5. Coarctation of the aorta. Lateral (*B*) retrograde aortogram. (*B*) A localized pinpoint constriction (arrow) lies just above the entrance of the ductus arteriosus (D) through which contrast medium passes from the aorta to the pulmonary artery.

Representative Cases

Case 6. Coarctation of the aorta. At age four months, this female infant was admitted in respiratory distress. There was a history of difficulty feeding and poor weight gain.

The blood pressure in both arms was 85/55 mm Hg and in the right leg 60/50 mm Hg. The neck veins were distended and the liver was enlarged. A grade III ejection-type systolic murmur was present maximal along the left sternal border. The femoral arterial pulsations were very weak.

Chest x-ray demonstrated caridomegaly, an enlarged left atrium and pulmonary plethora.

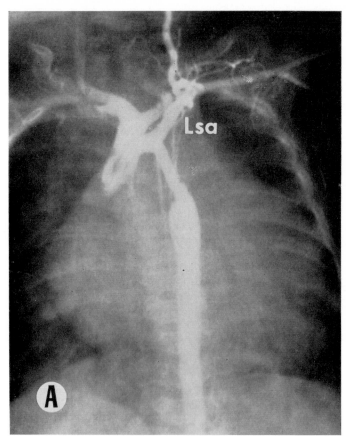

Figure 11-9. Case 6. Coarctation of the aorta. Frontal (A) countercurrent retrograde aortogram.

Right heart catheterization showed findings of a ventricular septal defect. A retrograde aortogram (Fig. 11-9 *A* & *B*) revealed a long area of narrowing of the aortic arch beginning just distal to the innominate artery and extending into the upper descending aorta. The aorta distal to this segment was markedly dilated. The left subclavian artery was enlarged. There was no evidence of an aortic-pulmonary shunt.

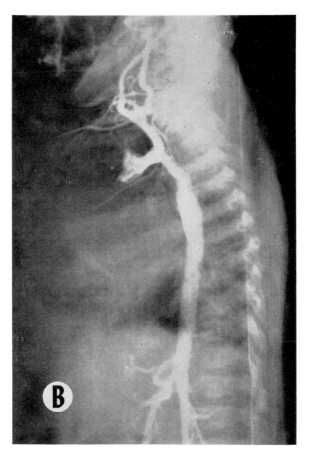

Figure 11-9. Case 6. Coarcation of the aorta. Frontal (*A*) and lateral (*B*) countercurrent retrograde aortograms. There is uniform narrowing of the aorta extending the length of the isthmus. Post-stenotic dilatation of the upper descending aorta is evident.

Representative Cases

Case 7. Coarctation of the aorta and aberrant right subclavian artery proximal to the aortic coarctation. This forty-seven-year-old woman was asymptomatic until one year prior to hospitalization when she developed dyspnea and fatigue. On physical examination, the right radial pulse was not palpable, and the left radial pulse was diminished. Pulses in both feet were markedly decreased. Blood pressure was 90/80 mm Hg in the right arm, and 125/95 mm Hg in the left arm.

Aortography (Fig. 11-10) showed a concentric constriction of

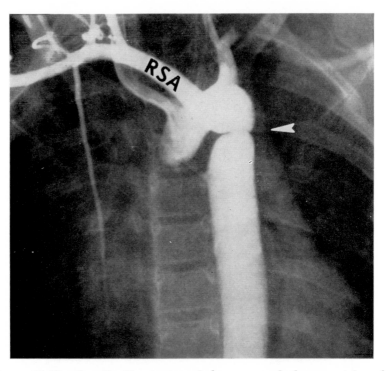

Figure 11-10. Case 7. Coarctation of the aorta and aberrant right subclavian artery. The right subclavian artery arises as the fourth branch of the aortic arch proximal to the site of coarctation of the upper descending aorta (arrow). Blood flow is in normal direction in the aberrant right subclavian vessel. This represents a postductal coarctation. (From J. R. Stewart, O. W. Kincaid, and J. E. Edwards: *An Atlas of Vascular Rings and Related Malformations of the Aortic Arch System.* Springfield, Thomas, 1964, Fig. 88.)

the aorta situated immediately distal to the origin of an aberrant right subclavian vessel. Following surgery, cerebral infarction occurred. Necropsy revealed that the coarctation had stenosed the orifice of the anomalous subclavian vessel. (Courtesy of Dr. James S. Stewart.)

Representative Cases

Case 8. Coarctation of the aorta and aberrant right subclavian artery distal to the aortic coarctation. This forty-three-year-old man complained of exertional dyspnea since childhood. At age twenty-eight, hypertension was discovered, but only in the left arm.

Blood pressure in the right arm was 110/76 mm Hg, in the left arm 180/90 mm Hg, and 100/70 mm Hg in both legs. Chest x-ray showed moderate cardiac enlargement, and there was rib notching present only on the left side, involving the sixth through ninth ribs. Aortography (Fig. 11-11 A-D) revealed a localized aortic coarctation distal to the left subclavian artery. An extensive collateral circulation involving the internal mammary and mediastinal arteries was demonstrated on the left side. On the right side, there was retrograde flow down the right vertebral artery filling the right subclavian artery, and subsequently the descending thoracic aorta distal to the coarctate segment. (Courtesy of Dr. J. H. Grollman, Jr.)

Representative Cases

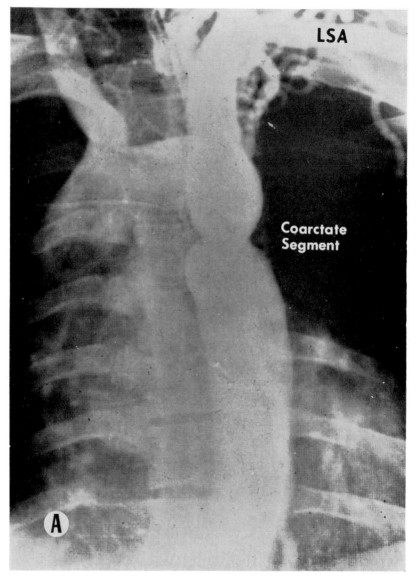

Figure 11-11. Case 8. Coarctation of the aorta and aberrant right sub-clavian artery. Frontal aortograms. (A) There is localized coarctation of the aorta distal to the left subclavian artery.

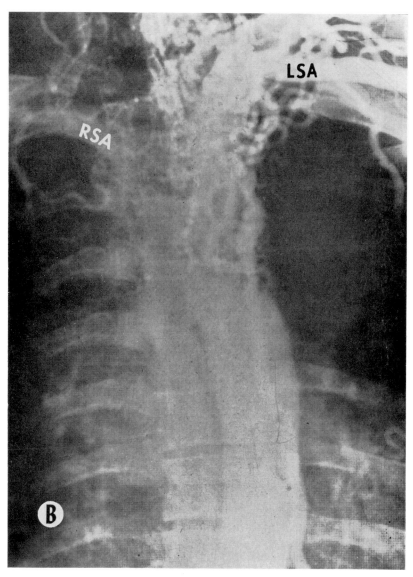

Figure 11-11. Case 8. Coarctation of the aorta and aberrant right sub-clavian artery. Frontal aortograms. (*B*) Two-and-one-half seconds after injection. The right subclavian artery is faintly opacified via multiple cervical vessels. Extensive mediastinal collateral pathways are present on the left side, with flow to the upper descending aorta.

Representative Cases

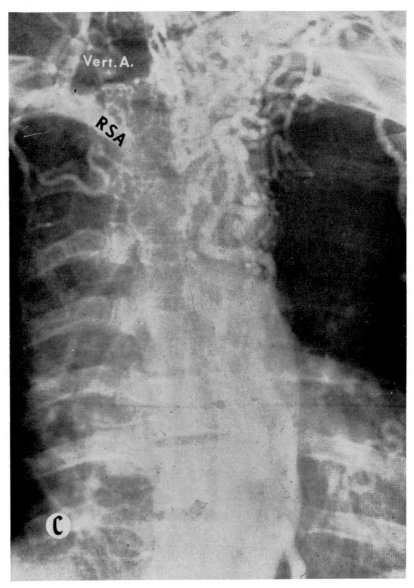

Figure 11-11. Case 8. Coarctation of the aorta and aberrant right subclavian artery. Frontal aortograms. (*C*) One sixth of a second later. The
right subclavian artery is further opacified receiving blood from the right
vertebral artery.

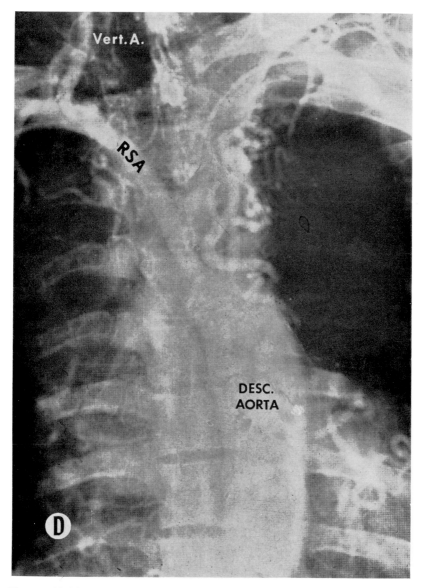

Figure 11-11. Case 8. Coarctation of the aorta and aberrant subclavian artery. Frontal aortograms. (*D*) Three seconds later. There is retrograde flow down the right subclavian artery to the descending aorta below the site of coarctation. (From J. H. Grollman, Jr., and J. W. Horns: The collateral circulation in coarctation of the aorta with a distal subclavian artery. *Radiology*, 83:622, 1964.)

Representative Cases

Case 9. Coarctation of the aorta and aberrant right subclavian artery distal to the aortic coarctation. This thirty-year-old teacher was hospitalized because of exertional dyspnea. Although the patient was right-handed, there was more strength in the left arm and hand. She gave no history of dizziness or fainting.

The blood pressure in the left arm was 140/90 mm Hg, 110/85 mm Hg in the right arm, and 120/100 mm Hg in the legs. Pulsations were very strong in the right carotid artery, and weak in the left carotid vessel. Pulsations in the legs and feet were diminished. Chest x-ray showed no rib notching.

Transseptal left ventriculography (Fig. 11-12 *A, B, C*) showed marked narrowing of the aortic isthmus. The right common carotid artery and the left subclavian artery were aneurysmally dilated. The left common carotid artery was small. All arose proximal to the aortic coarctation. Later films showed the right subclavian artery to fill by way of collateral channels in the neck. There was retrograde flow down the right subclavian artery opacifying the descending aorta distal to the aortic coarctation.

Selective catheterization of the right subclavian artery (Fig. 11-13) confirmed the huge abnormal flow down the aberrant right subclavian artery.

In spite of the large subclavian steal of blood, there were no symptoms of cerebral or vertebrobasilar insufficiency. (Courtesy of Professor W. Porstmann.)

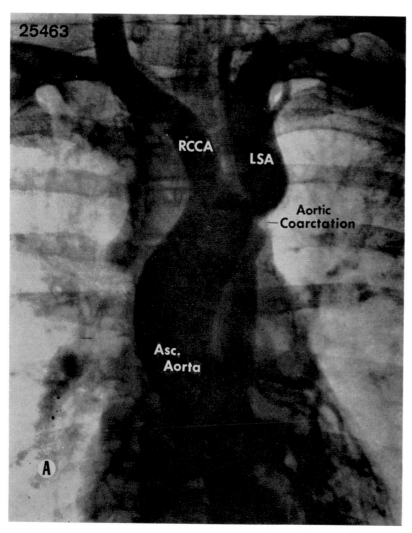

Figure 11-12. Case 9. Coarctation of the aorta and aberrant right subclavian artery. Frontal (*A*) and lateral (*B*) transseptal selective left ventriculograms show aneurysmal dilatation of the right common carotid artery, the left subclavian artery, and a small left common carotid artery which arise proximal to the aortic coarctation (arrow).

Representative Cases

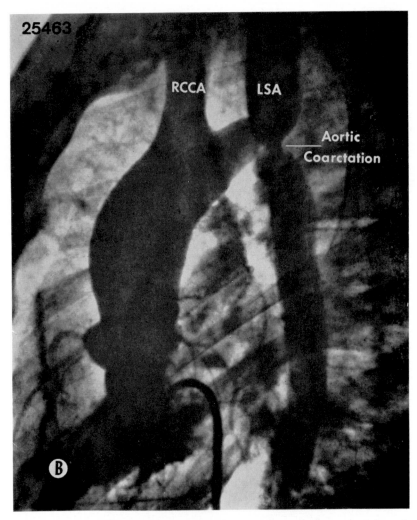

Figure 11-12. Case 9. Coarctation of the aorta and aberrant right sub-clavian artery. Frontal (*A*) and lateral (*B*) transseptal selective left ven-triculograms show aneurysmal dilatation of the right common carotid ar-tery, the left subclavian artery, and a small left common carotid artery which arise proximal to the aortic coarctation (arrow).

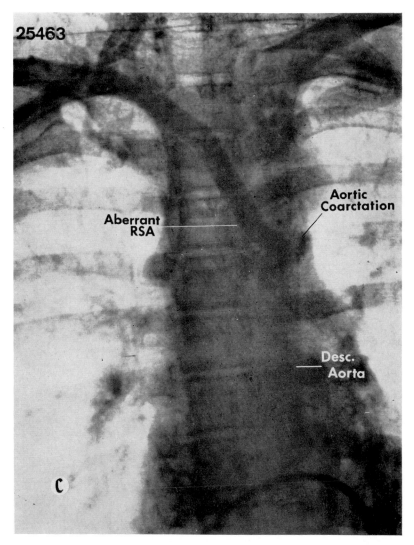

Figure 11-12. Case 9. Coarctation of the aorta and aberrant right sub-clavian artery. (C) Several seconds later, the right subclavian artery opaci-fies by collateral channels through its thyrocervical and costocervical trunks. There is retrograde flow down the right subclavian artery to the descending aorta. The right subclavian artery arises as the fourth branch of the left arch below the site of coarctation. (From W. Porstmann, K. H. Gunther, and W. Geissler: Aortenisthmusstenose mit atypischem abgang deider aa. subclaviae und bidirektionaler stromung in der a. subclavia dextra (A. lusoria).[1] *Fortschr Geb Roentgenstr Nuklearmed, 100*:465, 1964.)

Representative Cases

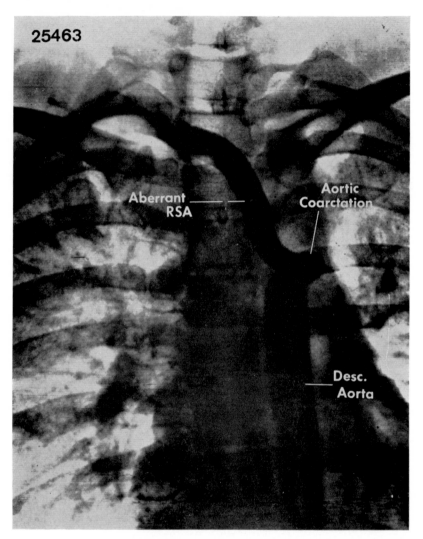

Figure 11-13. Case 9. Coarctation of the aorta and aberrant right subclavian artery. Retrograde injection of the aberrant right subclavian vessel with catheter tip in its first portion. There is a large retrograde flow down the right subclavian artery to fill the descending aorta below the site of coarctation. (From W. Porstmann, K. H. Gunther, and W. Geissler: Aortenisthmusstenose mit atypischem abgang deider aa. subclaviae und bidirektionaler stromung in der a. subclavia dextra (A. lusoria).[1] *Fortschr Geb Roentgenstr Nuklearmed,* 100:465, 1964.)

Case 10. Coarctation of the aorta proximal to the origin of both subclavian arteries. This thirty-three-year-old man gave a history of a heart murmur since birth. During childhood, he experienced epistaxes and headaches, and recently recalled episodes of dizziness during exercise. Otherwise, he was in excellent health and ignored recommendations to restrict his physical activities.

The pulse was 70. Blood pressure was 145/105 mm. Hg. in the right arm, 135/90 in the left arm, 145/110 in the right leg, and 130/100 in the left leg.

The patient was well developed with a muscular build. There was marked prominence of the carotid pulses. The heart was slightly enlarged with a sustained left ventricular impulse. There was a systolic thrill at the aortic area. A grade IV systolic ejection murmur was audible at the aortic area with radiation to both carotid arteries. A separate high-frequency murmur was present, maximal to the left of the fourth thoracic vertebra. The peripheral pulses were graded as follows (right/left): radial 2+, 3+; femoral 2+, 2+; carotid 3+, 3+; posterior tibial 2+, 2+; and dorsalis pedis 3+, 3+. The femoral and radial pulses were simultaneous and of normal quality.

Electrocardiogram revealed slight left atrial enlargement with left ventricular hypertrophy and strain.

Chest x-rays (Figs. 11-14, 11-15) showed left ventricular cardiac enlargement, prominence of the ascending aorta, and a soft tissue density in the left superior mediastinum suggesting an enlarged brachiocephalic artery.

Retrograde aortographic studies (Figs. 11-16, 11-17, 11-18) demonstrated coarctation of the aorta proximal to the left subclavian artery, with an aberrant right subclavian artery also arising distal to the coarctate segment. Cineangiograms disclosed a bicuspid aortic valve and slight aortic regurgitation. (Courtesy of Dr. Paul C. Kahn.)

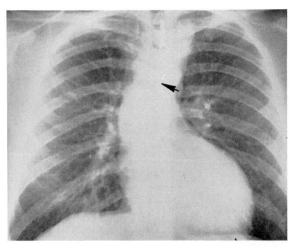

Figure 11-14. Case 10. Coarctation of the aorta proximal to origin of both subclavian arteries. There is enlargement of the left ventricle, prominence of the ascending aorta, and an indentation on the barium-filled esophagus (arrow). An opaque image in the left upper superior mediastinum suggests enlarged brachiocephalic vessels. (From Case Records of the Massachusetts General Hospital, Case 17—1973. *New Eng J Med*, 288:899-905, (April 26), 1973.)

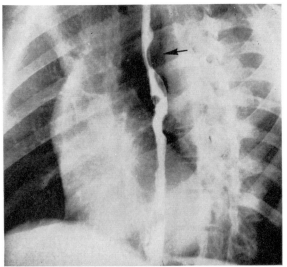

Figure 11-15. Case 10. Coarctation of the aorta proximal to origin of both subclavian arteries. Esophagogram, left anterior oblique projection, demonstrates a compression defect on the posterior esophageal wall at the level of the aortic arch (arrow). (From Case Records of the Massachusetts General Hospital, Case 17—1973. *New Eng J Med*, 288:899-905, (April 26), 1973.)

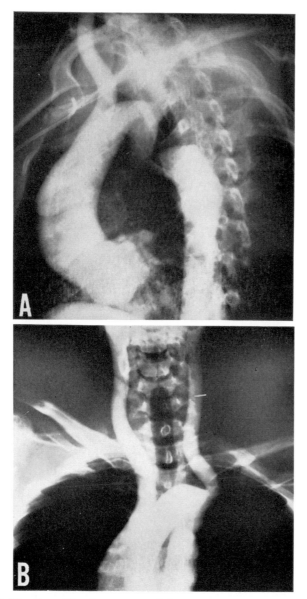

Figure 11-16. Case 10. Coarctation of the aorta proximal to origin of both subclavian arteries. (A) Retrograde aortogram, left oblique projection. There is coarctation of the distal arch, with visualization of enlarged carotid arteries, but no opacification of the subclavian vessels. (B) Frontal aortogram. The carotid arteries are markedly enlarged, without simultaneous filling of the subclavian arteries. (From Case Records of the Massachusetts General Hospital, Case 17—1973. *New Eng J Med*, 288:899-905, (April 26), 1973.)

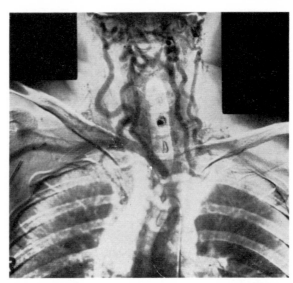

Figure 11-17. Case 10. Coarctation of the aorta proximal to origin of both subclavian arteries. Frontal aortogram, subtraction technique, several seconds later. Both subclavian arteries fill by retrograde flow through dilated cervical and vertebral arteries, with an anomalous origin of the right subclavian artery. (From Case Records of the Massachusetts General Hospital, Case 17—1973. *New Eng J Med,* 288:899-905, (April 26), 1973.)

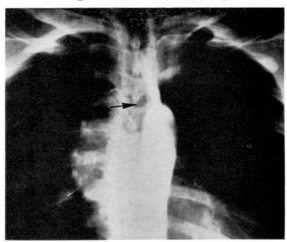

Figure 11-18. Case 10. Coarctation of the aorta proximal to origin of both subclavian arteries. Retrograde injection of the descending thoracic aorta. There is an anomalous origin of the right subclavian artery distal to the aortic coarctation (arrow). (From Case Records of the Massachusetts General Hospital, Case 17—1973. *New Eng J Med,* 288:899-905, (April 26, 1973.)

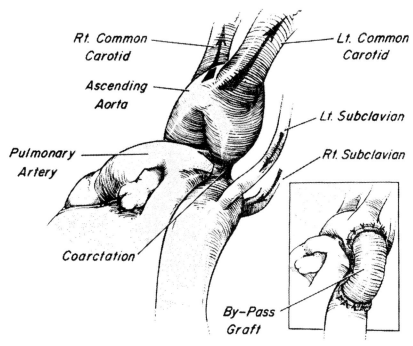

Figure 11-19. Case 10. Coarctation of the aorta proximal to origin of both subclavian arteries. Diagram of the coarctation and the surgical repair. Arrows show direction of blood flow in the subclavian arteries. (From Case Records of the Massachusetts General Hospital, Case 17—1973. *New Eng J Med*, 288:899-905, (April 26), 1973.)

Supravalvular Aortic Stenosis

Definition. A congenital deformity of the ascending aorta just distal to the origins of the coronary arteries.[4, 11]

Anatomic Types. Three anatomic types of supravalvular aortic stenosis may be encountered.[11] In the most common form, there is an hourglass deformity of the ascending aorta. In other instances, there is a simple fibrous diaphragm of the supravalvular aorta containing a single opening. Less commonly, there may be uniform tubular narrowing (hypoplasia) of the entire ascending aorta beginning just above the origins of the coronary arteries.[11]

Incidence and Clinical Significance. Supravalvular aortic stenosis is an uncommon form of obstruction to left ventricular outflow.[4] The anomaly may be familial. A peculiar facial appearance may be present with physical and mental retardation.[6] Clinically, the differentiation of this anomaly from aortic valvular stenosis and subvalvular aortic stenosis may be difficult. In some patients, there is an associated idiopathic hypercalcemia. There may be a difference of blood pressure between the arms.[4]

Chest Roentgenography. Chest roentgenograms usually show moderate cardiac enlargement without poststenotic dilatation of the ascending aorta.[4] There are no specific changes to distinguish this malformation from other obstructive lesions in the region of the aortic valve.[4]

Angiographic Features. Aortography will show the site of obstruction in the ascending aorta. Narrowing of the proximal portions of the brachiocephalic arteries may be demonstrated. Pulmonary arteriography reveals the associated peripheral stenosis of the pulmonary arteries present in some patients.

Representative Cases

Case 11. Supravalvular aortic stenosis. This nine-year-old girl was first seen in the cardiac clinic at age eight years with the complaints of mild headache, easy fatigability and mild exertional dyspnea. There was no history of syncopal episodes or congestive heart failure. Family history is of interest in that one cousin had undiagnosed congenital heart disease.

On physical examination, blood pressure in the left arm was 118/80 mm Hg, 90/70 mm Hg in the right arm, 95/70 mm Hg in the legs. The patient was well developed and well nourished. A palpable thrill was felt in the suprasternal notch that radiated into the carotid arteries. The pulse in the left arm was considerably stronger than the pulse in the right arm. There was a grade IV harsh, ejection-type, diamond-shaped systolic murmur best heard in the second intercostal space along the sternal border radiating well into the neck.

On cardiac catheterization, there was moderately severe obstruction of the pulmonic valve area with systolic elevation of pressure in the right ventricle. There was unusual restriction of manipulation of the catheter in the main pulmonary artery suggesting further constrictions of the pulmonary arterial tree. However, pulmonary angiography was not performed.

Retrograde aortography (Fig. 11-20) revealed severe obstruction in the region above the aortic valve with a hypoplasia of the ascending aorta. The coronary arteries were large and tortuous. The innominate artery and the left common carotid artery showed narrowing near their origins from the aortic arch.

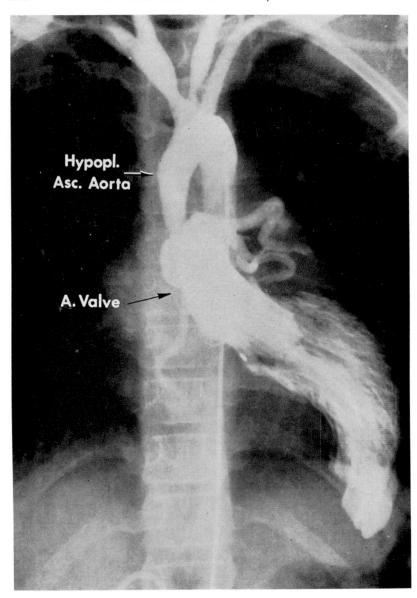

Figure 11-20. Case 11. Hypoplastic form of supravalvular aortic stenosis. Selective left ventriculogram. There is a tubular narrowing of the ascending aorta beginning just above the level of the origins of the coronary arteries which are enlarged and tortuous. The innominate artery and the left common carotid artery show narrowing near their origins from the aortic arch.

Case 12. Supravalvular aortic stenosis. This twelve-year-old girl was found to have a heart murmur during school examination. She was ,asymptomatic. The mother had coarctation of the aorta.

Physical examination revealed a well-developed child. Blood pressure was normal in both arms and legs. A faint systolic thrill was heard in the neck with a prolonged ejection murmur present along the left sternal border. The EKG was within normal limits. Chest x-ray was negative. The clinical impression was mild aortic stenosis.

Left ventriculogram (Fig. 11-21) showed a diaphragm-like constriction of the aorta at the supravalvular level.

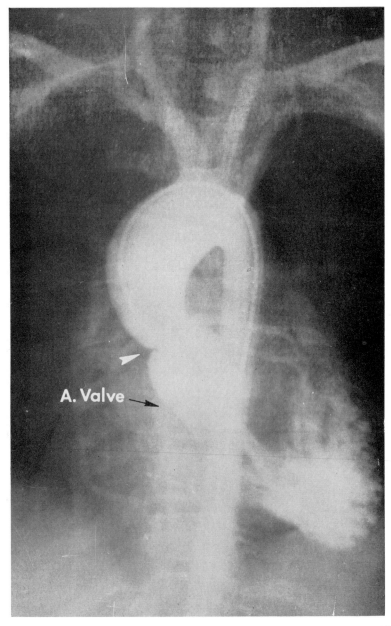

Figure 11-21. Case 12. Supravalvular aortic stenosis. A diaphragm-like constriction (upper arrow) is present at the level of the origin of the coronary arteries. Lower arrow indicates the aortic valve. The ascending aorta shows slight post-stenotic dilatation.

Case 13. Supravalvular aortic stenosis. This fifteen-year-old boy gave a history of a heart murmur since the age of five weeks and hypertension for ten years. Development and activity were normal, and the patient was asymptomatic.

On physical examination the boy was thin, but well developed. Blood pressure in the right arm was 155/100 mm Hg, 175/105 mm Hg in the left arm, 200/110 mm Hg in the right leg, and 195/105 mm Hg in the left leg. A loud harsh grade IV systolic murmur was heard over both carotid arteries. A systolic thrill was palpable over the upper sternum. Systolic and diastolic murmurs were present at the base of the heart. The electrocardiogram showed left ventricular hypertrophy and the chest roentgenogram revealed slight cardiac enlargement.

Right heart catheterization disclosed supravalvular pulmonic stenosis. Retrograde aortograms (Fig. 11-22, A & B) revealed an hourglass deformity of the ascending aorta at the level of the coronary arteries. Moderate to severe aortic insufficiency was present.

Representative Cases

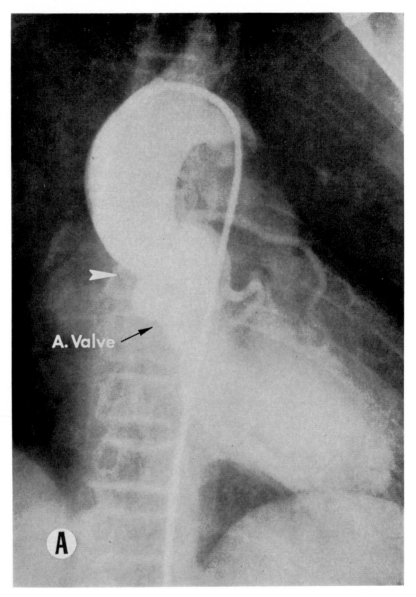

Figure 11-22. Case 13. Supravalvular aortic stenosis. Retrograde aorto-grams. (A) Hourglass type of narrowing of the ascending aorta (arrow). Moderate to severe aortic insufficiency.

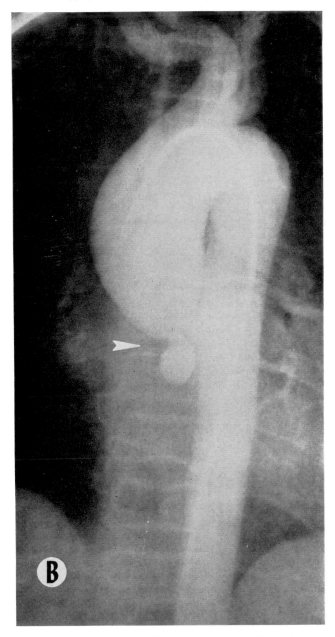

Figure 11-22. Case 13. Supravalvular aortic stenosis. Retrograde aorto-grams. (B) There is slight post-stenotic dilatation of the ascending aorta. Arrow points to stenotic segment.

REFERENCES

1. Case Records of the Massachusetts General Hospital. *New Eng J Med, 288*:899-905, 1973.
2. d'Abreu, A. L., Aldridge, A. G. V., Astley, R., and Jones, M. A. C.: Coarctation of the aorta proximal to both subclavian arteries producing reversible papillœdema. *Brit J Surg, 48*:525-527, 1961.
3. Drexler, C. J., Stewart, J. R., and Kincaid, O. W.: Diagnostic implications of rib notching. *Am J Roentgenol Radium Ther Nucl Med, 91*:1064, 1964.
4. Edwards, J. E., Carey, L. S., Henfield, H. N., and Lester, R. G.: *Congenital Heart Disease.* Philadelphia, Saunders, 1965.
5. Grollman, J. H., and Horns, J. W.: The collateral circulation in coarctation of the aorta with a distal subclavian artery. *Radiology, 83*:622, 1964.
6. Hurst, J. W., and Logue, R. B.: *The Heart.* McGraw-Hill, New York, 1970.
7. Klinkhamer, A. C.: *Esophagography in Anomalies of the Aortic Arch System.* Amsterdam, Williams & Wilkins, 1969.
8. Le Roux, B. T., Williams, M. A.: An unusual aortic coarctation. *Thorax, 23*:640-644, 1968.
9. Lopez, W.: Aortic atresia without significant hypoplasia of the ascending aorta. *Am J Roentgenol Radium Ther Nucl Med, 92*:888, 1964.
10. Perloff, J. K.: *The Clinical Recognition of Congenital Heart Disease.* Philadelphia, Saunders, 1970.
11. Peterson, T. A., Todd, D. B., and Edwards, J. E.: Supravalvular aortic stenosis. *J Thorac Cardiovasc Surg, 50*:734, 1965.
12. Porstmann, W., Gunther, K. H., and Geissler, W.: Aortenisthmusstenose mit atypischem abgang beider aa. subclaviae und bidirektionaler stromung in der a. subclavia dextra (A. lusoria). *Fortschr Geb Roentgenstr Nuclearmed, 100*:465, 1964.
13. Subramanian, A. R.: Coarctation or interruption of aorta proximal to origin of both subclavian arteries: report of three cases presenting in infancy. *Br Heart J, 34*:1225, 1972.

AUTHOR INDEX

SUBJECT INDEX